Prevention is better t

BREAST CARE
MANUAL
by
BRIAN H. BUTLER

REVOLUTIONARY, VITAL
NEW INFORMATION.
SAFE, SIMPLE, SELF-HELP
METHODS EVERY WOMAN
SHOULD KNOW & USE.

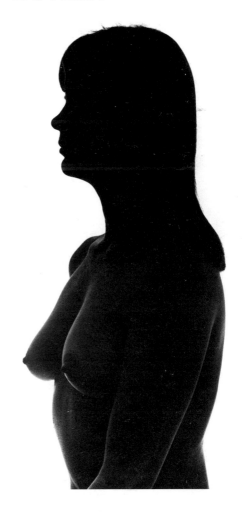

THIS PROGRAMME
SHOWS HOW
YOU CAN RELIEVE
tenderness,   soreness,
pre-menstrual pain,
heaviness, discomfort,
how you can help
reduce lumpy,
congested areas in
your breasts, and use
effective *preventive*
health care techniques.

First Edition: May 1993

British Library Cataloguing-in-Publication Data:

Butler, Brian Henry
  Breast Care Manual
  I. Title
  618.1

ISBN 0-9519279-1-4

Written, designed, illustrated, and typeset by the author.

Published by: T.A.S.K. Books,
P.O. Box 359A, Surbiton, Surrey, KT5 8YP

Printed in Great Britain by: George Green Litho,
Pitwood Park Estate, Waterfield, Tadworth, Surrey, KT20 5JL

CAUTION

The techniques suggested in this book are perfectly safe to use at any time.

They are not in any way offered, nor suggested as an alternative to any needed orthodox medical attention.

Most breast lumpiness, and most of the discomfort people have is simply due to lymphatic congestion, and will usually quickly be resolved by the use of the methods given herein. Appropriate manual massage enhances the body's own natural resources to cleanse itself.

The suggestions concerning health care with reference to exercise, clothing, diet, and apparatus, are made sure in the knowledge that they will improve the health and well-being of the reader when used in balance as suggested.

If you have any concern or anxiety whatever about your breasts, it is imperative you contact your medical doctor for their opinion without delay.

CONTENTS

CONTENTS

CONTENTS

DEDICATION

For women everywhere.
To the relief of anxiety and suffering
by using natural methods,
and where possible, the avoidance
of traumatic intrusions.

ACKNOWLEDGEMENTS

To Claire and Stephanie for their love, support,
and ideas, and painstaking proof reading.

With grateful thanks also to:

Dr. Mike Allen
Dr. Shamim Daya
Dr. Sheldon Deal
Dr. H. Keith Gooding
Dr. Bill Sagar

By the same author

Introduction to Kinesiology. 1990

Kinesiology for Balanced Health
Vol: I Basic. 1992
A TEXTBOOK ISBN 0-9519279-0-6

FOREWORD

When I first heard about this method of relieving breast lumps and congestion, I have to say I was more than a little sceptical. There seemed to be no physiological reason why such a thing should work. The notion that rubbing the outside of the thigh would have any effect on the breasts sounded strange indeed, in terms of Western medical ideas.

The first opportunity I had to observe this phenomenon was shortly after I had examined a woman of sixty-seven for breast tenderness. Her breasts were very lumpy and extremely sore. She said she even found it too painful to wear a bra, and turning over in bed was painful too.

The next day she experienced the methods explained in this book for relieving the pain and congestion. She came to see me again two days later, and told me that she felt a lot better. I then re-examined her breasts, and to my astonishment they felt much softer, and the lumpiness had virtually gone, and she expressed no feeling of pain or discomfort at all.

Had I not had the opportunity to examine her before and after, I frankly would not have believed that such a change was possible in such a short time. My sceptical nature still made me wonder if this was a "one off", so I took the opportunity to examine "before" and "after" with another patient. I again witnessed the same remarkable improvement. Having learned this technique, demonstrated by Mr. Butler, I intend using it when indicated in future

Naturally as a doctor, and a G.P., I heartily endorse Mr. Butler's frequent references to caution in respect of any breast problem. Delay is dangerous when there is a pathological problem, but no harm can be done by trying these techniques to see if they give relief, and change the lumpiness or discomfort, since they only take a few minutes to do and they may have a preventive value.

H. Keith Gooding, M.B.,Ch.B.,D.Obst.,R.C.O.G.
Maypole Surgery, Hook Road, Surbiton, Surrey. KT6 5BH

PREFACE

The procedures outlined in this book are simple. Please do not allow their simplicity to make you feel that they cannot be worthwhile. Some of the most beautiful truths in the world are the simplest. Some of the most wonderful things in life are the easiest to obtain. Having healthier breasts is simple to achieve.

We live in a complex, fast moving, technological age where new health products have to meet double blind trials and be held up to detailed scrutiny before they can be pronounced "good". This process is the one used to check the validity of drugs, and yet there is not one drug that does not have adverse side-effects which sometimes cause symptoms worse than the original problem they were used in an attempt to solve.

The method of rubbing a reflex on the side of the leg to relieve breast congestion may seem at first to be ridiculous. However, the proof of the pudding is in the eating as they say. All you have to do is to try these methods and see if they work for you. It would be wrong to say they work for everyone, but they certainly do work for the vast majority of women.

This technique has helped thousands of people, and it is time that it was public knowledge. Kinesiological techniques are one of the most powerful forces for prevention on the face of the earth today. There are many more you can learn about.

In view of the present day concern about breast congestion, and yes let's face it - breast cancer, certainly everyone will want to do all they can to keep healthy, rather than have to face the awful prospect of having to attempt a cure.

It is much easier to maintain a watchful eye on the stable door, rather than try to get the runaway horse back into the stable.

Remember: Prevention is better than cure.

INTRODUCTION

Breast lumps, breast congestion, and breast discomfort cause a great deal of concern for millions of women.

Statistics show that most biopsies taken of breast tissue show no abnormality in the cells. Most surgical intervention could be avoided by utilising the methods, and taking the simple, natural precautions and procedures given in this book.

Until recently, regular medical checkups were recommended, but now the emphasis has turned to self checks. Women are being told regularly to check the consistency and tone of their breast tissue, and to be aware of any changes.

Many changes in the breast are cyclical, and are linked to the menstrual cycle. These are usually the simplest kind to solve.

Most breast congestion, lumpiness, soreness, heaviness can be relieved in a few minutes, or after only a few sessions of two or three minutes duration.

If the congestion disperses using these techniques, you will have encouraged the body to do its own house cleaning in the most natural way.

Usually the long term lumps are due to the accumulation of waste materials. If these waste materials are not carried away by the lymphatic system, they form congestion. If this congestion is allowed to continue to accumulate over a long period, a cyst may form which becomes hard and uncomfortable. Even cysts can sometimes be systematically reduced in size until they are no longer to be found by using the suggestions in the pages which follow.

Remember, if in doubt, always consult your doctor.

AN AUTOBIOGRAPHICAL NOTE

One of the questions that I am most frequently asked, is how I first became involved with Kinesiology. Over twenty years ago, I was working in electronics, and was involved with computers. One day, my director telephoned me in my office. He wanted to ask if I could spare the time to look after a visitor from the United States for a few hours, and show him some of the sights of London.

As we drove around the city, I learned our guest was a chiropractor. This was something I had never heard of, but he explained it was somewhat similar to osteopathy, and was to do with adjusting bones to promote health, as well as help sore backs, and neck pains.

At the end of our day, I invited him to come home for tea. My elder daughter was writhing in pain on the floor. She had been having quite severe abdominal pains off and on for some years. After many visits to the doctor, various medicines and pills, nothing had helped to relieve this distressing gripe. It was said to be "growing pains".

My visitor asked if he may help. I was delighted, but could not think what he could possibly do for her. Within a minute, or perhaps less, she was smiling. The pain had gone. I was astonished, and asked him what he had done. He told me about Kinesiology, this amazing new discovery. He showed me the simple techniques he had used, and said it was safe for me to do it if she had a re-occurrence. It was eighteen months before she did. I worked on her as he had shown me, and she never again had a problem with her tummy pains.

Two years later, I was made redundant, and it seemed the ideal opportunity to go across to the United States and study Basic Applied Kinesiology, and bring it back to the U.K. and Europe. I have been practising and teaching Kinesiology ever since. Hundreds of health care professionals, both orthodox doctors, dentists, physiotherapists, and also complementary therapists, aromatherapists, chiropractors, masseurs, osteopaths, reflexologists etc., have attended my classes; as well as thousands of lay people who have wanted to learn the simple basics so they could help their family and friends enjoy life more, and enhance their own health and well-being.

The Author.

SOME TYPICAL ANECDOTAL CASES

Mr. R.D. is over the moon. A high powered executive who spends most of his business life jet-setting around the globe, he is neverthless very interested in natural forms of health care.

His wife had suffered a lot of discomfort with her breasts month after month, and he felt helpless and unable to do much more than attempt to console her when she was suffering. Then he discovered the breast decongesting techniques. He writes:

"My wife went for her regular check up with her gynaecologist recently, and during the session he checked her breasts for lumps. Upon finding one or two, he decided to take a scan and told her he would let her know the results later.

Naturally she was very alarmed indeed. Her distress was greatly heightened by the fact that she had to wait for the result. I asked her if she would like me to see if the reflex massage technique we used for monthly congestion would help at all. She felt that nothing would be lost by trying it, but I don't think she had much hope of it really helping.

Anyway, I started to massage the leg reflexes which were very sore for her. I had to work extremely gently at first. As the soreness diminished, so did the breast congestion. Within five minutes, they had disappeared completely and my wife could not find them. Needless to say, the diagnosis given by the specialist a week later confirmed that there was no problem.   **Mr. Roy.D.**

This wife and mother panicked when she found lumps:
I had been going for Kinesiology* sessions for some time, and had been getting a lot of benefit. The stiff neck and nagging pains in my back were virtually a thing of the past. The sessions made me feel so much better, that I continued to go regularly for maintenance care.

* See the section which explains the basics of Kinesiological health care.

I happened to mention to the Kinesiology* practitioner that I had just discovered lumps in my breast, and that I was extremely upset and worried about them. I told him that I had made an appointment to see my doctor, and he was pleased that I had. To my amazement, he asked me if I would like him to see if the lumpiness in my breasts would respond to a Kinesiological method of dealing with the problem. I have to say I was very sceptical.

But after only a few minutes treatment, he suggested I checked my breasts to see how they felt. I had noticed a sort of lessening in tension, and a lightness, but thought I may be imagining it. I felt my breasts thoroughly, and all the lumps had disappeared. I really couldn't believe it. The relief was incredible.

I did go to see my doctor just in case, and he told me he could feel nothing and there was nothing to worry about. He too was astonished to hear the story of the way they went.   **Mrs. S.A.**

A more serious success story:
I was telling a friend about the frightening experience that I had earlier on in the year. I have never examined my breasts before, but I noticed an irritating dry and itchy patch of skin on my left breast which had been bothering me for quite a while. However, on this particular morning, to my relief it had stopped being sore, but under the skin I could feel a large lump.

The next day I saw my G.P. who confirmed that he too could feel it. He suggested that I should see the surgeon who had operated on me the year before for a very difficult hysterectomy.

A mammogram and cytology was arranged and these tests revealed a 6cm mass which turned out to be non-malignant. We discussed what we should do next. He said that he would like to do a further needle test, and eventually remove the lump. I told him I would not have surgery, at which he expressed his horror, and said that we must discuss this some more.

* See the Appendix for more information about Kinesiology

I remembered being very impressed when I attended a weekend on Kinesiology many years ago. One thing in particular had stayed in my mind, and that was Mr. Butler's claim that there were techniques in Kinesiology which could sometimes get rid of lumps in breasts, although we did not see a demonstration of this on that occasion because nobody in the group had a lump. He had assured the group that it was possible. I was impressed that every other amazing technique he showed worked.

One of my closest friends died of breast cancer, and I always feel sad that I never had the opportunity to tell her about Mr. Butler and Kinesiology, because she went into hospital thinking it was just for tests, but they proved to be positive for cancer, and she came out having had a mastectomy.

Now was my opportunity to test Kinesiology out, so I made an appointment to see Mr. Butler. I showed him where the lump was located, and he could feel it as well. While he merely contacted the lump with a featherlight touch, he worked expertly using his fingers to massage specific places on various parts of my body. After he had finished working for a few minutes, he asked me if I could feel the lump. I told him I couldn't feel it.

About a week later, I saw my G.P. because I wanted to decide whether or not to have the second needle test which had been recommended by my surgeon. When my G.P. examined my breasts he said he could not feel any lumps, and therefore there would be no necessity for a further cytology test.

Six months later I saw a doctor in East Dulwich Hospital where I have regular oestrogen implants. He routinely examines my breasts, and on that occasion could not feel any lumps at all.

The dread for most women when they discover that they have a lump is of course the possiblity that it could be cancer. Due to fear, they act very quickly, and want the lump removed as soon as possible. Whilst urgent attention is required, the first option does not have to be surgery. In fact, for me it would never be surgery, I would always want to try a non-invasive method of addressing the problem first. **Ms. Susan D.**

An example of post-operative care using these methods:
I was treated successfully for breast cancer (lumpectomy, axillary lymph gland removal, chemotherapy and radiotherapy). The otherwise helpful and sympathetic doctors told me that I had simply to grin and bear the extremely uncomfortable mastitis I was experiencing - there was nothing they could do. Three years later it was still re-occurring, and causing me quite a lot of distress. Later I discovered the possible Kinesiology alternatives.

Two or three minutes of simple massage, and the 'hardness' vanished and so far, one month later, it has not returned. I'm certainly impressed and very grateful. **Suzannah E.**

Lady of sixty-four had "always" had tender breasts.
I thought that everyone's breasts must be tender. The state of my chest is not something I would think of discussing with other people, so I just put up with it. Looking back, I can't remember a time when they were not uncomfortable.

I have been going to yoga classes for years, and I have to keep reminding the teacher that I just cannot do certain movements because it is so uncomfortable to lie on my front, my chest hurts too much to relax into the postures.

I had been going to a Kinesiologist for some years, and greatly benefitted from the visits. I had had problems with my neck over the years, but although they were sorted out, I still went for my regular maintenance visits. As I lay down and turned over, I mentioned how sore my chest was. The practitioner asked me to turn over onto my back, and he worked with his fingers in firm massage up the side of my legs for just two or three minutes. He then asked my to turn over onto my front again, and I was astonished that all the discomfort had gone. **Mrs. J.A.**

ASPECTS OF BREAST SURGERY

Many women, and especially teenage girls, panic when they find some abnormality in their breasts. Because of the very real fears generated by so much publicity about breast cancer, some rush into surgery, that later tests may prove was unnecessary. Some women have been just for a check up, only to be recommended that some type of surgery be performed, "just in case" the problem was serious, but when the report comes back from the pathology lab., the excised lump was only fibrous tissue.

The vast majority of breast lumps are benign and harmless.
That is a medical fact. That does not mean that urgent action is not necessary, it is. When they locate some abnormality in their breast, far too many women try to ignore it, hoping it will go away. This is definitely not the approach to take. **Delay is dangerous. Never ignore any odd symptoms, even of itching, swelling, or any other changes.** But the need for urgent action does not mean the only option you have is surgical intervention.

The first action to take is to calm yourself mentally. Decisions made when you are worried, frightened, or upset, are rarely the best ones. Use the wonderful technique described in this book for Mental Stress Release, it will help you to look at the situation seriously, calmly, and in a balanced way. So if you feel there is a problem, take a few minutes to consider which course of action will achieve the best result for you. If the congestion, discomfort, or lumpiness can be relieved in one or two sessions using the methods shown in this book, there is very little chance of there being anything seriously wrong with your breasts.

However, do not let this stop you from seeking medical counsel to exclude possible malignancy, but while you are waiting for their opinion, you can try these techniques. The lumps may simply disappear after two or three sessions, which will give you great relief, and in consultation with your doctor, it may also avoid wasting the time of the specialists.

EVERYONE HAS CANCER CELLS

Abnormal or cancer-type cells are present in our bodies all the time. It is only when they start to multiply in an uncontrolled way, and produce areas of cancerous tissue that a problem begins to develop. In a healthy person with a vigorous immune system, cells which are in any way abnormal are taken out of circulation by the very wonderful self-healing mechanisms of the body. This is why it pays to keep as healthy as possible. See the section on nutrition and particularly the part on anti-oxidants.

Certain foods are known to have carcenogenic properties, like burnt and rancid fats found in some fast foods. The irritant oils and tars in tobacco smoke can cause cancerous tissue to form. It is also true that exposure to electro-magnetic radiation of certain frequencies like X-rays can cause cancer to develop.

The government of the United Kingdom has a national breast screening programme where women between the ages of 50-64 are offered the opportunity to have a mammogram every three years. A mammogram is a type of X-ray of the breast which is used in an attempt to detect abnormalities. There are some medical authorities who feel that by the time a lump is detectable on a mammogram, it has been allowed to develop far too long.*

There is also growing concern in some quarters that exposing the breast tissues to repeated X-rays could in the long term be contributing to the problem, in that each dose of X-rays is accumulative, and too many is definitely harmful.**

Another possible problem with having a mammogram on a regular basis is the force involved. The machine puts the breast tissue under about 40-50 pounds pressure, which can be very uncomfortable. Some studies suggest that if some tumours are manipulated forcefully, it can increase the chance of activating the spread of the cancerous cells to other parts of the body.**

* I Anderson et al (BMJ 1988; 297:943-48)   ** Dr. Swift, New England Journal of Medicine, 27-12-1991.

The finding of dormant, benign lumps, or cancer, may result in a decision to use surgery, and/or the use of radio-therapy, (more radiation) and chemotherapy, powerful drugs, which themselves may cause other cancers to develop. One study suggests that women whose cancers were detected by mammogram* have a shorter life expectancy than those women who do use regular self-examination. This suggests that regular self-examination may often detect problems earlier, and in a gentle way that does not aggravate the problem because of the use of force. Benign lumps are almost always best left alone, and not interfered with.

If anyone decides they do not want to have a mammogram for any reason, that is a decision they are entitled to make. It cannot be forced on you, although sometimes well-meaning people may unintentionally put you under psychological pressure to follow a course of action you would rather not be involved with. It is wise to explain to the doctor that you would prefer a physical examination, and if you show that you are someone who has studied the subject, they are more likely to respect your wishes.

The techniques in this book may be used with confidence. If you follow the directions exactly, no harm can result, and you will do some good. If a lump does not change there are several ortho-dox medical courses of action. One possibility is to have a bio-psy. This can involve using a fairly thick needle to remove a small amount of breast tissue under local anaesthetic. Since this may result in another lump forming some years later at the site of the incision**, thinner needles are now being used in some clinics which cause less local trauma to the breast. If surgery is suggested, ask if it is possible to take a less radical approach.

Before you agree to surgery, be sure you know exactly what is planned. Examine the consent form very carefully to ensure it describes in detail what is to be done. Check it does not give permission for more drastic surgery "should it appear necessary" during the operation, unless you feel and are sure it is in your best interests in the light of all the facts. Do not be pressured.

*P.Stomper & R.Gelman, Hematol Oncol ClinicN Am 1989; 3:611-40 **J.Dixon & T.John, The Lancet, 11-1-92.

SELF-EXAMINATION

It is a good idea to plan to examine your own breasts for any signs of abnormality on a fairly regular basis. It does not have to be something that dominates your thinking. It is best if you always maintain a happy, optimistic approach to your body. Remember, even if you do notice changes, most people's breasts vary in texture at different times of the month, and from time to time. It depends on circumstances like your current diet or stress levels, and this is nothing to be concerned about.

In order to establish a regular routine, keep a note of your periods in a diary. When you write it in, remember that after a period when your breasts are at their softest is probably the best time for self-examinations. When the change of life comes along, it is still important to continue to check your breasts regularly.

Choose a moment when you can take a relaxed look at yourself when you will not be disturbed by others needing to use the room. You will need a mirror, and good lighting is important. Make sure that the room is plenty warm enough so you will not feel cold with your clothes off. Take a few moments to calm your mind, (M.S.R. p.76) be positive, and mentally relaxed and happy.

Step 1.
Stand in front of the mirror, or sit if you prefer, with both your arms relaxed loosely at your sides. Lean slightly forward, and turn first to one side and then the other, all the time looking for any slight differences in size, shape, or changes in the contour, or any dimpling or puckering of the skin from the last time you checked. Then put your hands on your hips and press in to tighten your chest muscles, and check again.

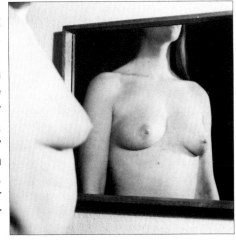

SELF-EXAMINATION

Step 2.
With both your arms raised so your hands are just above your head, look carefully at both breasts from different angles. Are there any changes since you last examined yourself? As you raise and lower your arms, notice whether the nipples go up and down by the same amount. (One is usually higher than the other this is normal.)You will have noticed if you had any discharge or bleeding from the nipples.

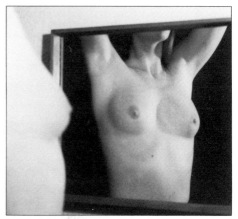

Step 3.
Lying down with another pillow under your right shoulder, and your right arm under your head, check your right breast with the flattened pads of the fingers of your left hand. (not the fingertips, the pads are much more touch sensitive.)

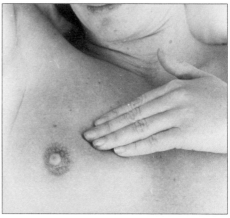

Imagine that the breast has six parts to check, four quadrants and the area around the nipples, and the "tail" which goes up to the armpit. First check the upper quadrant near the breastbone. Only use gentle, firm pressure, moving your fingers in small circles towards the nipple. Then check the lower inner quadrant. It is normal to find an area of quite firm flesh in this area, Then check around the nipple itself.

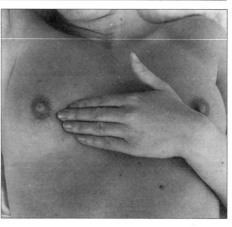

SELF-EXAMINATION

Step 4.

Now put your right arm by your side in a comfortable relaxed position, and check the outer two quadrants of your breast starting with the lower quarter, from underneath the bustline and up towards the nipple. Look at the nipple for any signs of cracking or change in shape.

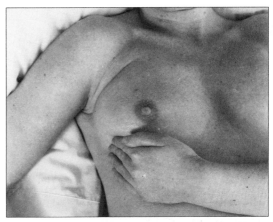

Step 5.

Then check your upper outer quarter in the same way starting near your armpit, and working down and across towards the nipple.

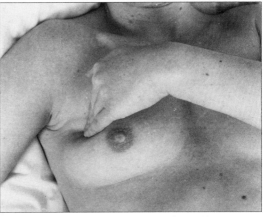

Step 6.

The last area to examine is the "tail" and up into the armpit. This is a muscular area, so it is   important your arm and shoulder are relaxed when you check it for lumps or any tenderness using the flat surface of all your fingers.

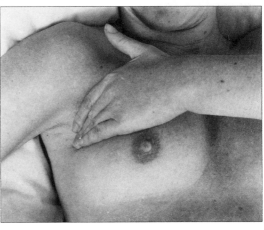

Then check the other breast in the same way. It is a fact that at least 40% of women have one breast larger than the other, and this is perfectly normal.

WHAT TO DO OF YOU FIND LUMPS

1. First of all, deal with your immediate reaction.
If you are unduly worried or upset, use the method suggested in the section on emotional and mental stress release. Sit down, touch your forehead as shown, and think through what you are actually feeling. Face your fears, and confront your concerns head on. Stare them out, so to speak, until they fade away.

2. Decide on a clear course of action.
If necessary with your fingers still on your forehead, plan what you will do, when, and how you will do it. Take your time.

3. Turn to the pages on relieving congestion.
Make yourself comfortable either sitting or lying down. Locate the area of lumpiness or congestion, and touch it gently while you rub firmly up the side of your leg finding the sore spots. (See pages 22-25) Do the sequence several times, see if you note any differences. If the lump goes away, so you cannot feel it, your breasts will feel more comfortable, maybe feel "lighter" and softer, and you will know that there is no serious problem.

4. Supposing it only gets smaller, but does not go away?
Plan to go through the procedure again later in the day, or first thing tomorrow. If possible find a friend, or a local Kinesiology practitioner, who is willing to work on it for you...and then ...

5. Make an appointment to see your doctor.
Remember, even if the lump or lumps do not go away using the techniques shown, 90% of all breast lumps are totally benign, usually being fibrous or cystic tissue. Only very rarely indeed are they cancer, and even then may not be a malignant form.

Unless your lump is clearly a problem, many G.P.'s may suggest you come back for a re-assessment next month straight after your period. If the lumpiness is still there, then they will probably refer you for further tests, or to see a surgeon for an opinion.

WHAT TO DO OF YOU FIND LUMPS

6. What if the doctor wants you to go for tests?

Do not be alarmed, it is better to be safe than sorry. Remember, at all times you are allowed to choose which treatments you will take, and it is important to take time to make the right decision. If the situation changes substantially, go back to your doctor and explain the progress you have made. This will give the doctor an opportunity to reconsider the need for further action. Everyone wants to reduce the cost of health care.

7. Continue the massage techniques.

While the month passes, or while waiting for your appointment at the hospital, work on yourself regularly. You can do no harm by continuing the gentle massage of your legs each day while touching the congested part of your breast.

8. Plan to start doing a a bowel cleanse.

Maybe you can decide to start a bowel cleanse using psyllium husks and gentle bowel strengthening and cleansing herbs from your health shop, to start getting your system as clean as possible. Bowel cleansing does not give you diarrhoea if done properly, and in accordance with the directions given on the packaging, by the health shop owner, or by your Kinesiologist.

9. If it goes away completely?

Celebrate! Then, after a telephone call to your doctor, and a visit if they request it to satisfy themselves that all is now normal , that may well be the end of the matter. No doubt you will be vigilant from now on, checking yourself regularly for any changes.

10. And if it does not go away completely?

It may be completely benign, and need no treatment at all. Needle aspiration or some surgery may be deemed necessary. Consider asking for a second expert opinion before proceeding, since you cannot undo any possible adverse effects of an aspiration, operation, chemotherapy or radio therapy.

RELIEVING BREAST CONGESTION

The technique for reducing chest congestion is simple and only only takes a few minutes, Amazing though it may seem, those tender, aching, sore, puffy, enlarged, painful, restricted feelings or being tender to touch, usually dissolve away in a short time.

Let us be very clear about this - it is never necessary to touch the nipples in the course of using any of these techniques. Let us also be very clear that although one of the techniques offered is called "breast draining massage", **there is never any need to massage the breast itself.** It is not necessary, nor is it desirable to massage the breast especially if they are sore, tender, or lumpy. **Massaging is only done around the breast.**

The techniques involve touching the sore areas of the breast with a feather-light contact. When any type of firm massage is indicated, this is only applied around the borders of the breast and on the upper chest, never on the breast tissue itself. It can either be done over clothing, or more effectively on the skin.

CAUTION: If you have any varicose veins on the outside of your leg, do not massage anywhere near them. In any event, do not overdo the massage of the leg. Ten to fifteen seconds on each area should suffice. You can always do it again after a while, or the next day.

It is only necessary to follow the steps shown on the next pages. Read the text carefully, then look at the pictures while you read it again. Then go through the three steps on yourself first. If you are going to ask someone else to do it for you, then you can show them the book, go through the steps with them, and tell them what you want them to do.

First, gently examine with the pads of your fingers for areas of the breast that feel in any way tender, lumpy or sore. When you find the exact point of greatest tenderness, you will then maintain contact with this area on the breast with the lightest touch all the time while you firmly massage the "reflex" described next.

The "Neuro-Lymphatic" reflex massage area which effectively mobilises the lymphatic drainage of the breast is located on the side of the leg. It extends from just below the knee joint, up the outside of the leg, (like the side seam of trousers) to the hip.

While touching your breast lightly with one hand, starting from just below the knee, massage a small area of this reflex at a time, up the side of the leg, until you reach the hip bone.

Each part of this reflex should be massaged with three fingertips. Place your fingertips firmly on the skin so that they will not slip off, and then without your fingers moving across the skin, rub in a rotating manner round and around. Some parts of this strip of lymphatic reflex will be more tender than others. You may want to pay especial attention to the most tender areas.

As you rub, if you are rubbing with the correct pressure, the amount of discomfort you feel on your leg will diminish slowly. This can sometimes takes longer than the ten-fifteen seconds spent on the other areas. Some really sore places may take up to half a minute for the degree of tenderness to begin to lessen.

When you get to the top of the leg, you can check your breast point again for tenderness. If it is gone, repeat the process from the knee up, while touching other sore areas, until your breasts are free of tenderness. Re-check the tender area on the breast, if all the areas of discomfort have now reduced or gone, fine. If the lumpiness is reduced but not gone, do it all again the next day.

Although you can do this for yourself, the results are often even more effective when the massaging is done by someone else. Perhaps ask a friend you trust to follow the procedures exactly as described. Usually the benefits will be felt straight away.

TO RELIEVE BREAST CONGESTION

Note carefully the position of the "Neuro-Lymphatic" reflex area on the midline of the side of the leg. Shown here on the left, they are in the same position on both sides of the body.

For effective lymphatic drainage of the chest, you can massage the reflex, and touch the breast through clothing, but it is much more effective when it is done with skin to skin contact.

For best results, massage this reflex up its entire length, section by section, in a rotating manner, while the pads of the fingers of the other hand are touching the congested or tender or areas on the breast. This usually has the effect of reducing lumpy, sore and congested areas of the breasts almost immediately. The effect will also continue working after you have stopped.

There is also a pair of reflex points on the back just below the tips of the shoulder blade in between the ribs. You will need to get someone else to rub these points for you, as it is virtually impossible to massage them properly yourself. It will be preferable and helpful for them to lightly touch your breast on the sore area at the same time.

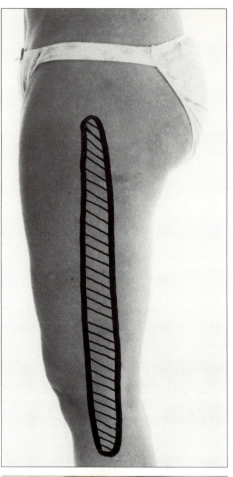

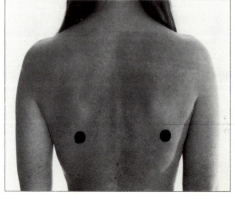

TO RELIEVE BREAST CONGESTION

STEP 1: Locate the areas of soreness or lumpiness.

STEP 2: Select the sorest point and touch it lightly.

STEP 3: While touching it, massage firmly the side of the leg.

Gently feel the different areas of the breasts to find where the most tender areas are. Check the sides, the areas around the nipple and around underneath the breasts. This should be done very carefully. When you find the most tender point, keep your fingers on it, and then......

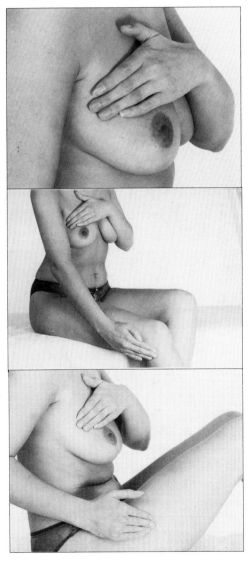

Start to rub the side of your leg on the same side with a firm circular motion. If you imagine where the seam of trousers would be on the side of the leg, that is where to rub. Start just below the knee, and rub each part firmly for about ten seconds then move up to the next point.

It is all right to overlap where you last rubbed. Pay particular attention to the parts of this leg reflex that are the most sore. If some places are very sore, start the rubbing gently and as the pain or discomfort reduces, then increase the pressure slightly. That is all there is to it!!

HOW DOES IT WORK?

No one really knows. The body still has many mysteries. Even highly qualified scientists wrestle with trying to unlock the secrets of Nature that have been written into the way we function as human beings. The electrical currents that continously flow through the nerve pathways in our bodies, produce complex associated magnetic fields. We are surrounded by clouds of electrical currents, which some peope refer to as the "aura".

The discovery of Kirlian photography, enables these electrical charges to be printed on a photographic plate, or paper. Eastern medicine regards the life force, or 'Chi, as being the vital spark that sustains life. Medical specialists are able to read some of the electrical waveforms that show that our brain is functioning normally, or that the heart muscles are responding properly to the electrical stimuli that make it beat in the rhythmic way it does.

The energy that extends from our fingertips for an inch or so, seems to be of a special nature. Touch healing does not invoke any external or supernatural force, it simply assists the body to normalise its own functions. There is apparently some electrical significance in touching the breast while rubbing the leg.

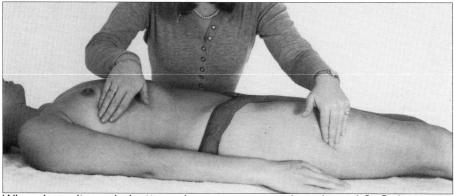

Why does it work better when someone else does it? Quite apart from the fact that someone else is caring for our concerns, there is "healing" in the touch from a friend, whether a comforting arm around the shoulders, or a mother's touch on her child's pain.

THE ELECTRICAL PART OF US

Acupuncturists say that the 'Chi travels in pathways called the Meridian network. Each of our organs draws part of its energy from a Meridian it is connected to. For each organ to work at its best, the energy has to flow freely and without blocks. Healthy breasts need a clear, unimpeded flow of these energies.

This Kirlian photograph shows how the energy which surrounds out of our fingertips can be captured on film. The size and the shape of this energy varies according to how we feel, and the level of our vitality. People skilled in reading these photographs can sometimes gain useful insights.

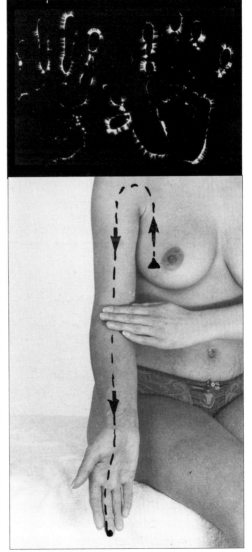

The energy meridian, or energy pathway which is related to the breasts is shown here. This vital energy flows one way in the direction of the arrow. It starts about one inch outside the nipple on both sides of the body, and runs down the centre of the arm to the middle finger of each hand.

Brushing very lightly over the skin in the direction shown will encourage the energy to flow. It is a bit like brushing ones hair, this lines up the energy fields, and encourages them to stay in balance. This is something to do a few times after a shower, or when doing daily exercises.

CHEST LYMPH DRAINING MASSAGE

The more efficient the flow of blood and lymph to any part of the body, the more healthy that area will be. The health of the upper chest will be improved by massaging the tissues in the directions shown on the picture below. Massage the upper chest in the direction of the arrows with gentle but firm pressure using a little massage oil. This will encourage the lymphatic flow towards the main draining ducts and to the axillary glands in the armpit.

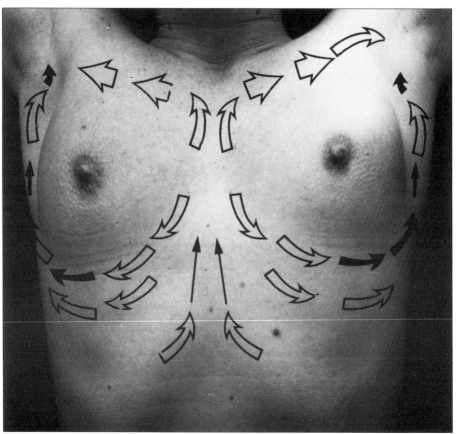

This is a massage technique that you can do effectively for yourself. However, if you know another person who is interested in massage work, they may be able to achieve even more effect for you than you are able to doing the massage yourself.

CHEST LYMPH DRAINING MASSAGE

This technique is ideal for a preventive regime of regular massage. If the procedure shown here is practiced once a month or so, the chances of a build-up of congestion in the breast tissue will be greatly reduced. If congestion is prevented, more serious problems cannot ensue. The first stroke is across the upper part of chest towards the armpit.

The massage is best done in a flowing way with your two hands following each other in a way that they overlap each other. Here you see the direction and extent of the travel of one hand. Start very lightly at the beginning of the stroke, and then gradually increasing the pressure slightly as you go along the line of massage. It should not be heavy pressure at the end of the stroke, but it should be quite a bit firmer than at the start.

In this picture, you see that the other hand has followed on, by starting just a short distance after the place where the first hand started, following exactly the same line as the first stroke towards the armpit. Again, at the beginning of the stroke the pressure is light, and gets a little firmer all the way along the line of the stroke. It is nicer if you come off the skin with a gradual reduction of the pressure at the end of the stroke.

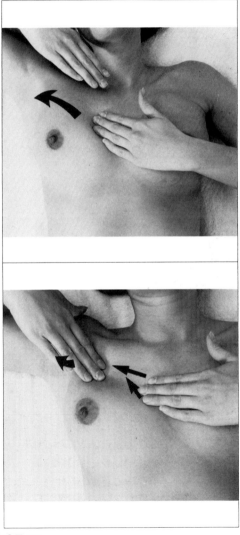

CHEST LYMPH DRAINING MASSAGE

Each stroke overlapping the last a little bit, means that the strokes get shorter until the tips of the fingers or the heel of the hand almost reach the armpit. Then you begin the next stroke at the place where you originally started. This helps gently to move the lymph flow towards the lymph glands which act as "drains" in the armpit.

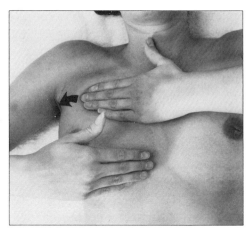

It can also be done in the opposite way working out from the armpit medially with each stroke towards the axilla longer than the previous one. This causes a vacuum which draws the lymph from the centre line of the chest towards the ducts in the armpit. From here the lymph is drawn into the main lymphatic ducts which are found behind the collar bone.

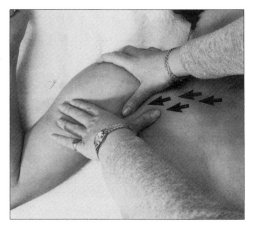

The same technique is also used under the breasts up into the armpit. Start at the breastbone with your fingertips and/or your thumbs moving with a steady firm pressure, around and underneath the actual breast tissue. If it is not found too uncomfortable, a little extra pressure in the space between the ribs is also beneficial.

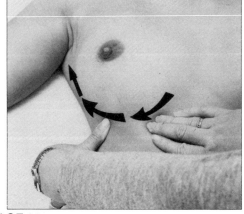

CHEST LYMPH DRAINING MASSAGE

Then following through around and under the breast, work up towards the armpit in a series of sweeping, flowing strokes using the thumb or fingers.

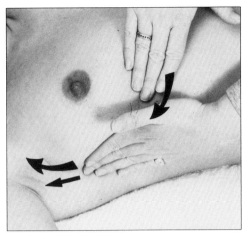

Each stroke following the other as before, gradually moving around the chest and up just below the armpit itself. It is better not to massage the actual armpit, but allow the suction in the lymph system to take care of that area.

Another useful technique is to put the middle three fingers of each hand in the soft spaces between the ribs either side of the sternum, or breastbone.

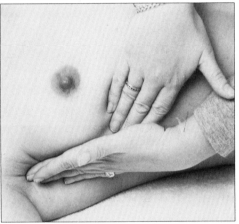

When you have them located, anchor your fingertips on the skin, firmly massage outwards and also towards the middle, back and forth in a series of short movements.

This stimulates other Neuro-Lymphatic reflexes which help keep other areas of the chest tissues in tone.

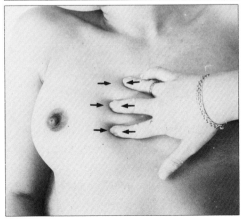

An ideal time to do this, as part of your daily routine, is after the bath or shower.

THE LYMPHATIC SYSTEM

The job of the lymphatic system is to feed and clean the tissues of the body, and that includes the breasts. There are about eight pints of blood in the body, and its job is to carry oxygen and nutrients to the tissues, and to remove the carbon dioxide and other toxins. As the blood, pumped by the heart, flows into the smallest blood vessels called capillaries, some of the plasma of the blood escapes into the surrounding tissues.

Plasma is a non-cellular fluid which contains nutrients, It bathes the tissues where the large red blood corpuscles cannot go, and feeds and nourishes them as well. This inter-tissue fluid becomes lymph which also contains white cells. These white cells, called lymphocytes aid in the protection of the body from infection.

There is approximately twice as much lymph as blood. Simply put, its job is to feed and clean the body tissues where the blood cannot go. There are about twice as many lymph vessels as blood vessels. This vast network of tiny lymph vessels flow against gravity towards and into the lymph glands located in various parts of the body. We are most concerned here with the ones which are in the armpit, called the axillary glands.

The heart pumps the blood around the body, but the lymph has to rely mostly for its flow on pressure in the system created by everyday movements. This flow can be greatly enhanced by certain exercises. The main lymph glands are located in parts of the body where there is a high amount of activity. As it flows up the body, it is prevented from flowing backwards by flap valves.

At the end of its journey, as it enters the main draining ducts near the neck, its flow back into the blood stream is assisted by the movements which are involved in breathing. It is because lymph flow is so important, that we are paying special attention in this self-help manual to skin brushing, chest massage with oil, exercises and breathing, all of which encourage lymph flow.

THE LYMPHATIC SYSTEM AND THE HEALTH OF YOUR BREASTS

In the diagram below, the position of the main lymph glands is shown. The ones we are most concerned about in maintaining healthy breasts, are the ones in the armpit called the axillary glands, and the main ducts at the base of the neck. The lymph glands are filters which prevent the passage of germs into the rest of the body.

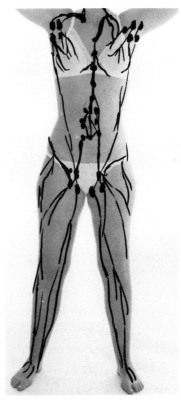

The white cells in lymph also attack and destroy any invading organisms and thereby this helps contain the infection and prevent it from spreading into other tissues. The lymph fluid also removes other toxic matter, including dead cell debris.

If there is too much toxic matter, the lymph system can become overloaded in certain areas. If this happens, then parts of the system can become inflamed, swollen, or even painful. When glucose is burnt in the tissues to provide energy, the by-products of this metabolism are then transported by the lymph to the blood, and then excreted.

Gentle lymphatic drainage massage can assist lymph flow, and increase its effectiveness in clearing the system of toxic wastes. It is vitally important that the lymph flow is not restricted and not impeded in any way. So we will look at ways to keep the lymph flowing to ensure that the breasts are kept clear of toxins.

SKIN BRUSHING

Some interesting research has been done into what happens when the skin is stimulated by massage. The effect it has on the internal workings of the body is much greater than previously realised. It has long been known that it stimulates the blood supply, but it also has a profoundly beneficial effect on the organs, muscles and the nervous system. The effect we are most interested in here, is the stimulation of the lymphatic system.

Our bodies are made of cells which have a limited life span. They die off and are continuously replaced by new cells. When the cells die, they are broken up into tiny parts by specialised organisms which are then drawn into the lymph vessels where they are further broken down by the white corpuscles. This house cleaning process is continuous, but it can get stagnant, clogged up, and then problems can ensue.

The more efficiently the lymphatic system is working, the cleaner and better fed are the tissues it bathes. Drainage of the breast tissues is especially important. The breasts are external to the body so to speak, and subjected to restrictions and pressures by clothing which can inhibit lymphatic flow. This is the reason we address the need for bras to fit well in the next section.

The cells of our skin are also dying and being replaced all the time. If these dead cells are removed from the surface of the skin by gentle brushing, the skin can "breathe" more easily. The skin is the largest organ of elimination, and needs to be kept "clean".

Dry skin brushing's most important benefit to breasts is that it can help to accelerate the flow of lymph through the tiny vessels, and into the main lymphatic drainage ducts. From the large lymphatic vessels, the lymph is drawn into the bloodstream so that the toxins can be excreted through the kidneys. Inner cleanliness produced by dry skin brushing will show externally in the healthy glow of the skin, and in improved overall health.

HOW TO DO DRY SKIN BRUSHING

Skin brushing is well worth the short period of time it takes to do. Some authorities have suggested that just five minutes of skin brushing, can be the equivalent of an extra half an hour of exercise. If you do your exercise programme every other day, do the skin brushing routine on the days you do not do your usual exercises.

What sort of brush do I need?
Pure bristle brushes are fairly expensive, but they are really the only ones to use. Natural bristles do not scratch or abrade the skin. Cheaper brushes made of plastic or synthetic fibres may damage the surface of the skin which defeats one of the main objects - a healthier, clearer skin. If you can get one which has a wooden handle which you can attach and detach, you will find it better for doing your back.

After you have been skin brushing for some time, you may want to use a stiffer brush. Find one which has natural vegetable fibres, maybe coconut, which will last a long time. It is more important to get your skin well used to being brushed regularly before you try using stiffer types of brush.

When shall I do it?
To do dry skin brushing, your skin needs to be dry! Do not do it when you are hot and perspiring after exercise. If you are going to exercise as well, skin brush first. It is probably best to do it just before you plan to have a bath or shower. Then when you have finished brushing, you can wash off the dusty waste matter you have loosened from the surface of the skin straight away. First thing in the morning is probably the preferred time.

Anytime is fine, but you may want to avoid doing it just before you go to bed, as it can be quite stimulating, and make it difficult for you to get off to sleep. The important thing is that it becomes an enjoyable part of your programme of health care routine.

HOW TO DO DRY SKIN BRUSHING

Note Bene: Only brush in one direction - towards the heart.

Start at your feet, brush up the inside of your legs up to the centre of your torso by the tummy button or navel.

Then start again at the feet, this time on the out-side of the legs, sweeping up the side of the legs across the hips finishing again near the navel.

Then sweep up the back of the legs, up over the hips, around to the front, and up to the navel. All of these three described here can be repeated 1-4 times.

Then start at the back of your hands, brush towards the centre of your chest over the upper surface of your arms. Then brush from your palm to the arm-pit along the underside of your arm.

Then brush from the side of your hips up each side of your body to the armpits and then as much of your back as you can reach from under and behind the arms around to your navel.

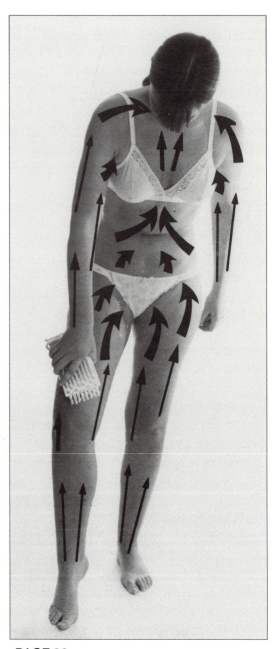

PAGE 36

WAYS TO IMPROVE LYMPH FLOW

1. Move around regularly.

Nowadays so many people have a sedentary lifestyle. Pressures at work mean that breaks are sometimes few and far between. The lymph system is not working at its best when we are sitting down, especially with the legs crossed as so many people do.

Take a break every hour for just a minute or two, even if it is only walking to the end of the corridor and back, or walking up and down a short flight of stairs. The time spent will be well rewarded with increased concentration and working efficiency. It is possible to become so engrossed in the work, especially if one is in front of a computer screen, that time goes by so fast, and before we know it, we have not moved for two or three hours.

The same applies when driving long distances. When planning the journey, build in time for periodic stops every hour or so. Get out, have a brisk walk for a minute or three. You will drive more alertly and safely as a result.

2. If you have a hectic, moving around job, rest regularly!

Stop for a minute or two each hour to give the body a chance to restore its internal equilibrium. There is nothing so refreshing as a change of pace. All systems get an opportunity to normalise.

3. Encourage lymph flow while you are asleep.

Lymph relies mostly on muscular action to promote its flow. If you sleep soundly, you will not move around a great deal.

Put some wooden chocks under the legs at the foot of your bed so that the foot of the bed is about an inch, or an inch and a half (3-4cm) higher than the bedhead. In this way, gravity will assist the flow of lymph all night while you are asleep, and your body will be more rested, and cleaner when you wake up. It can also help lymph flow a little more if you are able to organise it so that your bedhead is pointing towards the North Pole.

FREEING UP THE LYMPH CHANNELS

No. 1. AVOID TIGHT CLOTHING

The health of any part of the body depends upon the free flow of body fluids through the tissues of that part. A law of physics states that a very small restriction in a tube through which liquid is flowing causes a drastic reduction in the amount of fluid that gets through. So a tiny change in the size of the lymph vessels due to undue pressure, can mean a big reduction in lymph flow. Impeded lymph flow can result in congestion.

Bras that are too tight restrict the flow of blood and lymph in the chest area. In an attempt to get adequate support for their breasts, some women tend to buy a brassiere which fits quite tightly around the torso. Other women who might feel a little self-conscious about the size of their breasts, may buy a smaller size in the hope of making their breasts appear smaller. Some bras may shrink after many washings, and the reduction in size may not always be noticed.

Putting the bra strap on the tightest possible hooks and eyes in order to get support makes matters worse. It is far better to rely on the shoulder straps to take the weight. Whatever the reason for doing so, it is never a good idea to have a tight band around your body, and particularly not around and under your breasts.

Also, many bras are under-wired around the base of the cup. This metal may slightly affect the delicate electrical currents that control the distribution of lymph. In the space between the fifth and sixth ribs under the breasts, are important reflexes which affect the lymphatic drainage of the upper chest.

Even the constant slight pressure from the underwired bra that was too tight may also slightly inhibit the free flow of lymph by causing an over-stimulation of the lymphatic reflex which tends to reduce the flow. This adverse effect is lessened if the material used to gain the extra support is inert, like plastic boning.

WEAR GARMENTS THAT FIT WELL

The pictures below illustrate the problems described on the opposite page. Breast congestion, discomfort, and concern about lumps make it sufficiently important to pay attention to the way your bra fits. Regularly invest in new garments when the old ones have lost their shape or elasticity. It is false economy not to spend money on, and time selecting this most important piece of clothing, for it can negatively affect your overall health.

When the bra strap is done up too tightly, it can cause quite a considerable reduction in the flow of body fluids in the upper chest. Look at your back view and see if there is a bulge. If there is a red mark, or weal when your bra is removed after some hours of being worn, it is too tight.

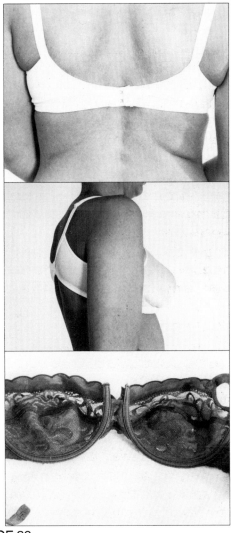

If the shoulder straps are too short, the bra rides up at the back, and cuts into the skin in the front of the chest in the space between the fifth and sixth ribs. After hours of wear, this can be very uncomfortable and it can inhibit the lymphatic flow in the upper chest.

Some bras which are under wired with a metal band, if worn too tight, may slightly affect the breast lymphatic reflexes. The continual friction from the metal bar, although it is covered with fabric, can over-stimulate the reflexes, and may also have a slightly negative effect on the lymph's electric control circuits.

WEAR THE RIGHT SIZE & TYPE BRA

An astonishing fact came to light in the course of research for this book. Professionally trained lingerie staff in large stores were consulted. They were unanimous in their opinion that from 70% - 90% of all the ladies who consult them are wearing the wrong chest size, cup size, or in some way the bra they are wearing is not fitting correctly.

This almost unbelievable statistic means perhaps many millions of women could be in a position to enhance their appearance, health, and well-being, simply by buying a more appropriate bra. It appears that many women have a conflicting image of themselves and their bra size that is just not correct. It may or may not have been correct at one time, but our bodies change shape and size as we mature. This fact needs noting well.

In a practical assessment, a young woman went to a well known department store, and asked the trained lingerie expert to give her advice and help. An hour later, she left having purchased four makes of bra, all of which were a different size! They ranged from 34A to 36B, but all were a suitable and comfortable fit for her. This can happen because the manufacturers of brassieres have different views and approaches towards how best to make a garment to fit the breast.

The moral of this story might be best expressed in the words of one highly trained lingerie lady: "Would you ever even consider buying a pair of shoes without trying them on? If not, why even think about buying a bra straight off the counter of your local department store?"

The skilled expertise you need is usually available in your local department store. It will pay you to ring up and enquire whether they have specially trained assistants in the lingerie department. You may want to ask which company has trained them, as they will obviously be slightly biassed towards their own products.

TEN POINTS ON BRAS TO CONSIDER

The experts consulted all agreed on the main important points concerning the selection, purchase, wear, and care of this most important piece of ladies attire.

1. Start young.
If the breasts are supported as soon as they develop, then un-due stretching of the upper chest tissues can be reduced. It is also best to face the issue early, and get used to the idea, to avoid embarassment later.

2. Avoid having pre-conceived ideas.
Be willing to be flexible about what size chest and cup you are, or you think you should be. Have an open mind, be willing to revise your opinion of yourself, even if the size that fits you best does not match your usual size. Never buy one that is too tight.

3. Get professional advice.
Seek counsel from a professional who has been properly trained by manufacturers. They will have the experience necessary to give you sound advice on the type of bra you need to help you to enjoy optimum breast health, and enjoy a nice appearance.

4. Always try it on before buying.
Make it a rule never to buy a bra without first trying it on, and preferably with the expert help of someone there who is trained to take an objective view. It does not pay to be shy in this area of life. Of course, if you know which one fits best and you definitely have not changed in size or shape since you last bought one, then buying one "off the shelf" is time saving.

5. Plan to take your time.
Plan your visit to the store so that you are not rushed. Then you can take your time to try on several different makes of bra, compare chest sizes, and cup shape and size, and examine them to find the one which really suits your body shape best.

TEN POINTS ON BRAS TO CONSIDER

6. Sizing guidelines.
One manufacturer gives the following guidelines:
To find your bra size: Measure under the bust in inches. If the number of inches is an odd number add 4, and if it is an even number, add 5.

     I.e. If under bust = 29" + 5 = Bra size 34
         If under bust = 32" + 4 = Bra size 36

If the calculation comes out so that it is in between two sizes, say 37, then buy a 38. it really is vital that it is not too tight for you.
To help find your best cup size, measure round the fullest part of your breasts, and compare it with the under bust measurement.
   If it is the same it indicates an A cup may be best for you.
   If it is 1" more = B cup; 2" more = C cup, 3" more = D cup
   If it **is** 4" more = DD cup, and 5" more = E cup.

7. Avoid under-wired bras for all day use if possible.
If you find the right bra that fits really well, you may not need the under-wiring. Also, you can ask whether they stock some of the makes that use plastic boning instead, and these are better, so long as they fit you properly.

8. Wash your bras by hand.
That may sound like a chore, but this way you will not use water that is too hot. If bras are washed in water that is too hot, and for too long, they lose their elasticity, and the support they give will deteriorate quickly, which is a waste of money.

9. Buy new ones regularly.
Like any other garment, a bra has a limited life. It is too easy not to notice that they have seen better days. After a certain length of time, you know they will need replacing, so do it. Resist the temptation to put off buying a new one. Do it today!

10. Sports Bras.
If you exercise regularly, (please do!) - buy a special sports bra.

IT ONLY WORKS IF YOU USE IT
Any information is of value only when it is put to use.

The information in this manual, if put into practice on a daily basis, will make a very great difference to your overall health and especially the health of your breasts.

At the beginning of this manual, it was stated that the methods for relief of breast congestion, and all the other techniques offered would be simple, and easy to do. We hope that you are finding this is true, and there is more to come.

Most exercise bikes finish up in the garage.

Most diets are started and abandoned several days later.

Most New Year resolutions get forgotten by January 6th.

Changing lifestyle habits is not easy - it takes a lot of effort.

Why are we so resistant to change? It is fear of the unknown. We know what it is to be like us, just the way we are not. What we might be like or have to face if we change we do not know, and that can frighten us subconsciously into avoiding change. Better the devil you know ..... or is it?

The average person has 2.4 colds a year, eats junk foods, spends too much time watching television, rarely exercises, does not look for ways to improve life, and slowly deteriorates.

Do you want to be average? No! Of course not. Then swim upstream, and enjoy life more than ever before each day.

Success breeds success, nothing succeeds like success. So be successful. Be a winner. The publishers would like to hear of success stories about how people have used this knowledge to improve their health, vitality and well-being, and tell others too.

FREEING UP THE LYMPH CHANNELS

No 2. AVOID THE USE OF ANTI-PERSPIRANTS

The sweat glands in the armpit are vital to upper chest health. They are a direct route out of the body of many nitrogenous and other toxic waste products. They also allow the skin to "breathe". It is very important for the sweat glands of the body to be able to release perspiration. Perspiration evaporates from these glands even when the armpit feels dry. This evaporation causes a flow of fluids to replace the amount of perspiration that evaporates.

Perspiration contains materials which attract bacteria which multiply rapidly in the warm, damp environment of the armpit. Unpleasant armpit odour is largely due to these bacteria. It is not necessary to seal the sweat gland ducts with varnish, or glue like substances in order to prevent odour. It is only necessary to use some type of deodorant that kills off the offending bacteria, this neutralises any odour which may come from the sweat itself.

Ordinary perspiration, and sweat from exertion does not smell strongly in a fit and healthy person. It is only when a person is cleansing toxic matter that any odour is noticeable. Another good reason to exercise regularly!

Perspiration which is caused by nervousness, mental tension, or fear, often has a more distinctive odour. This odour helps make us consciously aware that we are nervous, and signals to others that we are under tension whether they realise it or not. This odour can be neutralised with an appropriate deodorant. The formulations vary from one manufacturer to another, no deodorant suits everyone, It is important to find one which suits you.

Maybe, you could plan only to use a deodorant which contains anti-perspirants when you know that you are going to exert yourself a lot, such as at a dance, or when you are likely to be nervous, as when on a first date or job interview. Otherwise, avoid anti-perspirants wherever possible.

USE ONLY NATURAL DEODORANTS

You may want to check out your local stores and health food shops for types of deodorant which are based on natural herb formulas, which may be just as effective for you.

This close-up of the skin of the armpit shows clearly the area where the skin must be allowed to breathe. Anti-perspirants tend to seal up the pores with lacquer or other substances that dry, and leave a coating over the skin's pores that prevents sweating. You can buy natural deodorants that do not contain these substances.

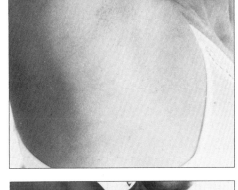

Avoid using anti-perspirants as much as possible in order to allow the moisture from the sweat glands to evaporate freely. Only use them when needed for special occasions. Be sure that you thoroughly cleanse the area after use, to open up the pores again.

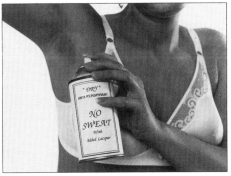

There are many different types of deodorant on the market. Some of them are made from pure herbal sources, which only contain natural substances. It is necessary to select one which suits you. Each person's bio-chemistry is slightly different, so pick one that works for you.

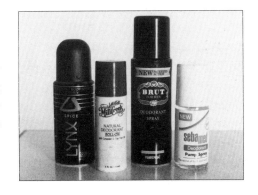

FREEING UP THE LYMPH CHANNELS

No 3. GET REGULAR EXERCISE

Our lymphatic circulation depends a great deal for its overall efficiency upon the muscular movements of the body. Of course, we all move about quite a lot in the course of each day. As we walk about, stand up and sit down, go up and down stairs, the lymph vessels are being massaged by the muscles.

It seems that in the realm of exercise, most people are in an "all or nothing" mode. There are those sports buffs, who may be seen jogging every day, or going off to the gym or sports club. They get lots of exercise, perhaps too much for some who may be overtaxing themselves without realising it.

On the other hand, probably the vast majority of people almost never take any form of regular exercise. They will find any excuse not to exercise. Lack of exercise is certainly one of the causes of poor health and lack of vitality. It is a factor in breast health which should give every woman an incentive to exercise regularly.

Possibly the best natural regular exercise is to take a brisk walk twice a day. Many people who commute have this opportunity each day. If you normally travel by bus, you may like to think about leaving a little earlier each day and consider walking a few bus stops up the road. Similarly in the evening, perhaps get off the bus a few stops from home, and walk the rest of the way.

Undoubtedly, the finest form of exercise to promote lymphatic drainage is the use of a rebounder. The flap valves in the lymph vessels close up every time you jump, and open as you go down, pumping the lymph effectively. These mini-trampolines offer a wonderful way to get the valuable lymphatic exercise you need for health in the convenience and the privacy of our own homes. No need to travel to the gym or club, or buy or wear special clothes, apart from a good sports bra.

REGULAR EXERCISE IS ESSENTIAL

Doctors agree that regular moderate exercise is essential to attain, and to maintain optimum health. You do not have to be an exercise buff, or use up hours in exercise for it to be effective.

Brisk walking, swinging both arms is a very good way to get exercise, and it stimulates the flow of lymph effectively. No equipment is needed, and the benefits are many. It is worth working out how to spare the time to walk regularly. Check with your doctor before taking up any strenuous exercise.

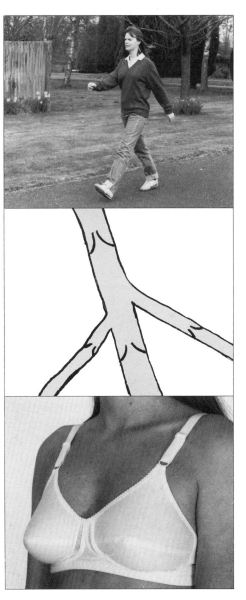

Along the length of the lymph vessels, there are one-way flap valves, which prevent the lymph from draining down the body.This causes the lymph to rise up the body through the lymph glands to the lymphatic ducts in the base of neck, thence back into the blood-stream.

A Sports Bra is a vital piece of sports equipment This has a very specific job to do while you are exercising and you need a specialised garment designed for this purpose. Do not be tempted to exercise in your day wear bra. Your breasts need the extra support from a sports bra.

REBOUNDING, BEST FOR BREASTS!

Rebounding not only pumps the lymph through the system most effectively, there are many other side benefits to be gained. Not the least of which is that after a short period of seven or eight minutes, those who regularly work out on a rebounder find their spirits lift. They find they feel more positive and creative as well as being invigorated by the exercise. Check first with your doctor that it is all right for you to embark on a gentle regular exercise programme. Then here are some useful guidelines to help you derive the most enjoyment out of your rebounding sessions. Don't forget to wear a special sports bra!

1. Start gently. Rebounding is a very time/effort effective way to exercise. Start by gently jogging for maybe one or at the most two minutes. Do time yourself so as not to overdo it.

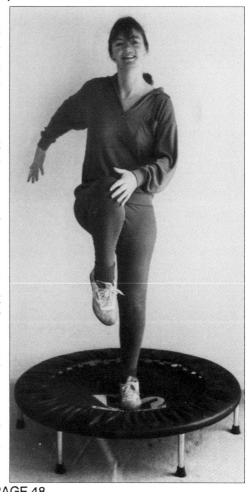

2. Use music. Good music is uplifting and healing. Different rhythms will inspire you to use different movements.

3. Buy a good book on the subject which will give you new ideas, and much more useful information on rebounding.

4. Increase your time every other day until you are doing at least ten minutes in one of your sessions. **Don't overdo it.** Do not exceed your maximum "exercise heart rate". Find it by subtracting your age from 180.

5. Enjoy. Regular rebounding produces a joyful feeling. Your fitness improves, and so does your sense of well-being.

SIMPLE WAYS TO FIRM THE CHEST

These two very simple exercises that are really easy to do will help to strengthen the muscles that support the breasts. A good time to do them perhaps, is while you are jogging gently on your rebounder, or after you have done your skin brushing routine.

EXERCISE No. 1
With your elbows bent, press your palms together firmly and maintain that pressure, while you bring your hands **slowly** from waist level to above your head as high as you can stretch, and then downwards in a smooth continuous movement bring your hands back down to your navel again.The two most important points here are to maintain a steady pressure between your palms, and to do the exercise slowly. There is no benefit in doing it quickly.

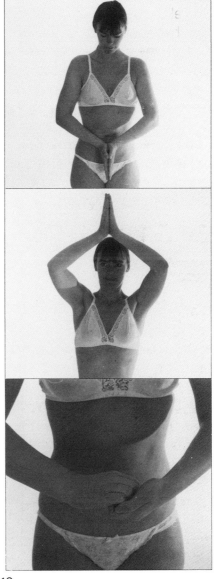

Exercise No. 2
This is very similar, except you interlock your fingers and maintain a pressure as if to pull your hands apart, while you slowly raise your arms from your waist, past your face and up above your head as in exercise No. 1.

Continue the sweep as high as you can, then smoothly start to come down again to waist level. These two excellent exercises help tone and strengthen some of the main muscles that keep your breasts supported, and also help increase the lymph flow.

FREEING UP THE LYMPH CHANNELS

No 4. Learn to breathe diaphragmatically

One of the three main ways in which the lymph is pumped around the lymphatic system is by the action of breathing.

Each time you breathe in, lymph is sucked from the large lymph vessels in the upper chest into the lymphatic ducts. These ducts are the "main drains" of the lymphatic system. They are at the end of the system, just before the lymph gets forced back into the bloodstream. At this point, the lymphatic fluid contains the maximum amount of debris and toxic material which the body wants to get rid of.

Each time you breathe out, lymph is forced from the lymphatic ducts into the main veins leading to the heart. Once the lymph is in the blood, the waste products are filtered out by the kidneys, passed to the bladder, and excreted in the urine.

Most people do not breathe effectively. If only the upper chest and the rib cage rise up and go down with each breath, the lungs are only being partially filled with life-giving oxygen.

Diaphragmatic breathing, or belly breathing as it is sometimes called, fills the lungs much more efficiently and with much less effort. It might seem like hard work to start with, but the more you practice, the easier it becomes.

Practice breathing slowly and deeply. Do not overdo it, or you may hyper-ventilate and get a bit dizzy. Once you are breathing slowly and deeply, cause your abdomen to extend as far as it will go out with each in-breath, keeping your upper rib cage still.

As you breathe out, compress your abdominal muscles under your rib cage so that the air is forced out gently and completely. Changing the habit of a lifetime is not something you will achieve overnight, it takes a lot of practice.

BREATHE DIAPHRAGMATICALLY

Learning to breathe diaphragmatically really pays off in terms of greater health and increased sense of well-being, more energy.

The lungs are like bellows which are narrow at the top and wide at the bottom. Chest breathing leaves the greater volume of the lungs unfilled with air. It may feel easier, but it leaves the body with a lack of life giving and health producing oxygen.

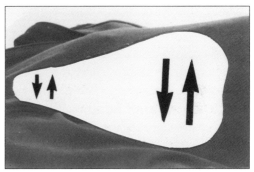

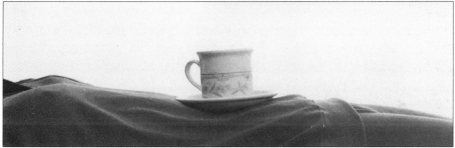

Diaphragmatic breathing, otherwise known as belly breathing, fills up the lungs more fully with each breath. You will find you have more energy, feel more alive, and have more stamina for the day, and for your evenings too. This gently massages all of our internal organs.

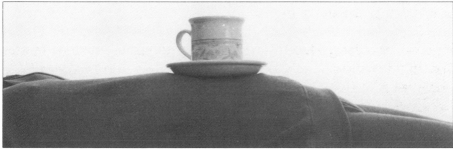

Practice belly breathing with a small weight, like a cup or mug on your abdomen and watch it rise up and down as you breathe diaphragmatically. Do this in the morning before you get up, and in the evening before you go to sleep, and you will instill a new good habit.

DRINK PURE WATER AS A HABIT

No 5. Drink pure water every day

Our bodies are made up of over 75% water. Water is being lost all the time by evaporation through the skin, and out through the bladder as urine. This water needs to be replaced.

One function of the water we drink is to cleanse the body. If we drink water that contains impurities, those impurities have to be sorted out, and then excreted. Regrettably some impurities stay in the body and accumulate.   For instance, lead from water pipes, mercury from industrial wastes, and other highly toxic substances are not always excreted, but remain in the body to cause different types of health problems.

Due to the reckless manner in which water is used by industry and by the general public, it has to be recycled artificially. While the water companies do their best to filter out particulate matter, and remove or destroy organisms that could cause disease, it is impossible and uneconomic for them to purify the water so that all the mains supply is high quality drinking water.

We do not need ultra pure water to clean cars, water lawns, or fill swimming pools. But, we do need ultra pure water to drink.

Water is the only substance we take into our mouths in quantity that does not require digestion. Tea, coffee, colas, lemonade, and fizzy drinks of all kinds, contain numerous ingredients which have to be digested by the body. The digestive system needs also to be cleansed, and to be given a rest. So drink water.

Drink six to eight glasses of pure water daily. It is a good idea to buy some sort of filter, further to clean and purify the water from the tap that you drink and cook your food in. Jugs are good, and plumbed-in types are usually better. Someone you know will know someone who sells them. They are worth the money in terms of enjoying long term a healthy water supply.

PLAN TO DRINK PURE WATER

It is really worth while for the sake of your long term health to make sure that the water you drink is as pure as you can reasonably make it. Yes, it costs money, but it pays handsomely!

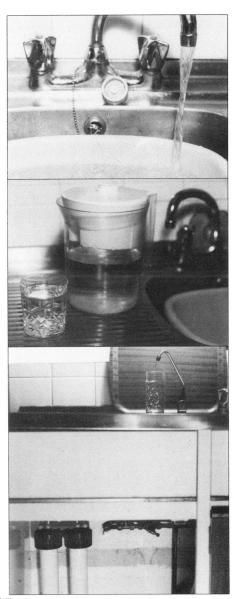

The water that comes out of the tap is a compromise. The cost would be prohibitive to purify all water to a very high standard, and it is not necessary. Tap water may contain some very low level impurities, like drugs and chemicals, the long-term effects of which are not known.

One method of ensuring that the water you drink and cook with is of a higher standard than the tap water, is to purchase some kind of filter jug. These are tedious to fill up regularly, but they really do improve the quality of the water. Be sure regularly to change the filter as directed. Sales of bottled water have also rocketed in the last few years.

More expensive initially but much cheaper in the long run is for you to install a plumbed-in filter. The one shown, nearly anyone can fit on a D-I-Y (Do-It-Yourself) basis and is a double filter. One part is ceramic, it filters out very small particles; the other is granulated carbon to remove more of the dissolved chemicals and gases.

THE NUTRITIONAL PART OF US

There is no doubt we cannot live long without food. Unhappily many people are suffering starvation in the world today. In the Western world, we have what appears to be a super-abundance of food. The shelves of our supermarkets contain an awesome array of foodstuffs. We are spoiled for choice.

Yet, in a way many of us are malnourished, even if we eat three meals a day. You cannot have clear skin, good muscle tone, and yes, healthy breast tissue, if you lack nourishment. So much of what we eat does not contain the life giving vitamins, minerals, or energy we need for robust health. Great arguments about this rage back and forth. Some say you can get all the vitamins and nutrients from the food, others say you cannot. Who is right?

One thing is certain, most people do not feel very well. They lack energy and drive, have the regulation three colds and one bout of 'flu per year, are pretty much constipated, fed up, and do not sleep particularly well. But when you ask them how they are, they may reply, "Fine." They are not, of course, but that is the socially acceptable superficial answer.

A recent survey of how people in the U.K. spend their money in the average supermarket was a shocking revelation. The first ten items were, in order of millions of pounds spent annually:
1. A make of cola drink. 2. & 3. Two makes of washing powder.
4. A brand of coffee. 5. A type of cat food. 6. Crisps. 7. A brand of whisky 8. A type of tea bag. 9. A Margarine 10. A dog food.

It is interesting to note that these are all individual brands of the item concerned, not all brands of colas or teas! The top amount spent on each item started at £350 million annually, and went down to £120m. If you add all the other makes of these types of product, one wonders what the total expenditure would be!!

What is also interesting is that these things are not basic foods!

NUTRITIONAL OR SLOWLY TOXIC?

One important fact is emerging from many areas of research into nutrition. Those who are properly nourished, and have a really balanced intake of vitamins and minerals in their diet, are much less affected by pollution, radiation and other external toxic influences. It really does pay to spend a little time educating ourselves about the basic dietary needs of the human frame.

Some experts say all disease has part of its root in malnutrition. It is getting harder and harder to buy food that is as nutritious as it is cosmetically attractive. Things are dressed up to look really delicious, but do they contain the vital substance we need to be healthy rather than just survive?

One way which helps is to eat a good variety of fresh vegetables every day. It is amazing how many people say they do not like vegetables. A balance of cooked and raw vegetables eaten as part of our daily fare, provides much of the fibre, vitamin, and mineral content we so badly need. It is quite important for each of us to find out what is the best proportion of cooked and raw foods that suits us best. We are all different. What is fit for the goose, is not always suitable for the gander. A lot of raw food and roughage, especially bran, does not suit some people.

Manufactured, processed foods contain much less of these vital elements of sound nutrition. Regrettably they also contain some of the thousands of "permitted" chemicals and additives. Some experts have said that we are in the process of experiencing the biggest, most far reaching, totally uncontrolled experiment in human nutrition ever conducted.

Nobody knows what the effects will be long term. Pollutants from food, water, and the air we breathe is like having a time-release poison seeping into your system. This slowly but surely has had a general affect on the nation's health, and will wear down our vitality and resistance to disease if nothing is done to change it.

FOODS BEST KEPT TO THE MINIMUM

Foods that are difficult to digest, or those that make the organs work harder, are best kept to the minimum. You may want to take a fresh look at those things we commonly eat and drink which stimulate the body, but leave really toxic residues behind.

That is not to say anyone has to become faddy about diet. It simply means giving thought to balancing what we eat. There are some simple guidelines which if followed will keep your body and in particlular your breast tissues in better general health.

1. Commercially prepared foods are not as good as fresh.
Virtually all commercially prepared foods are either processed, frozen, contain additives of some sort, or are generally not as nutritious as a similar thing you might prepare yourself from fresh ingredients. Tastier perhaps, but not so nutritious. The food industry would argue this point strenuously, and although this is a generalisation, it holds true for most things.

2. Avoid fatty, fried and "fast" foods as much as possible.
There is a lot of evidence to suggest that consuming a lot of fatty foods clogs up your body's systems. Some suggest it may be linked to some forms of breast cancer. It is not just a question of the dreaded cholesterol. Your body has to make quantities of that, no matter how much we eat in our food. It is much more a question of rancid and saturated fats. Fats solid at room temperature being harder for the body to digest and handle.

3. Dairy products
The pasteurisation of milk destroys much of its natural goodness and makes it much harder for the body to digest. Many people are sensitive to milk because they were weaned onto it too early in life, before their digestive systems were sufficiently developed to handle it. Hard cheeses also fall into this category. It is better to avoid margarine than to avoid butter. Most people seem to handle and benefit from yoghourt and cottage cheese very well.

FOODS BEST KEPT TO THE MINIMUM

4. Alcohol
Great in moderation! People who drink small amounts of alcohol quite often seem to enjoy better health and longer lives.

5. Carbonated drinks
Carbon dioxide is a narcotic. It is toxic to the body, that is why we breathe it out. Filling the stomach with water into which large quantities of CO_2 have been dissolved means there is one more burden for the body to cope with. Mixed with alcohol, they affect the body more rapidly.

6. Sugar and sugar substitutes
Sugar is bad for you. We do not need it. The body will make the glucose it needs from complex foods. We certainly do not need to consume quantities of sugar each day. It is only partially true that it gives you energy. What we are not told by those who wish to sell it to us, is that it can cause energy lows, hypoglycaemia, mental depression, aggression and hyperactivity, and more.

A trial period of largely cutting sugar from the diet in American prisons resulted in fewer attacks on warders and less fighting among the inmates. Can we learn from this? Sweeteners are unnatural substances, often made out of coal tar products. Far better to re-educate the taste buds or use a **little** honey, or that real luxury, maple syrup.

7. Caffeine and Chocolate
Caffeine is in many drinks, and there is often more than 85mg in strong coffee, and some in cocoa too. Chocolate can cause congestion problems, and is best kept as an infrequent treat.

8. Smoked foods, pickles, additives and preservatives, salt
There is a high chemical content in many of these products, and some contain a lot of vinegar and sugar. Excessive salt is often connected with circulation, heart, and kidney problems.

FOODS FOR BREAST HEALTH
We are what we absorb from what we eat, drink and breathe.

THE VITAL IMPORTANCE OF FIBRE IN FOODS
An interesting comparative study was made between a group of people who lived in one of the world's major cities, and a group of similar size in an African country. Without going into lots of detail about the study, the important finding was that many people in the city group had some form of bowel cancer and none in the group of Africans.

The reason for this, it was concluded, was that the Africans were eating entirely unrefined foods with lots of ground grains, fresh vegetables and fruit. The city dwellers on the other hand were eating a diet which consisted of mostly refined foods, processed "white" grains, very few vegetables, and little fruit.

Many people in the West think that all they have to do is add some bran to their diet and all will be well. This is not so. Bran is an irritant, and may well contribute to problems if it is consumed unwisely. Psyllium seed husks are much better at providing gentle bulk if that is needed from time to time.

Raw or cooked?
Ensure you eat some raw foods every day in or as near their natural state as possible. Some say eat everything raw, and that certainly does not suit everyone. Each person needs to find the ratio of raw to cooked foods that suits them.

Diets
Faddy or restrictive diets, fat free, low cholesterol, high fibre, strict diets and relaxed diets, no one diet works for everyone. Eating sensibly is what works best. It is what you do every day that counts. A once a week treat does no harm.

Buy food that will go bad, and eat it before it does.
In a more natural world, all the food we consume would itself be

FOODS FOR BREAST HEALTH

in a state of decay. The moment a cabbage is picked from the field, its nutritious values begin to degrade. A fish, once it is out of the water begins to deteriorate, and it is only because of our modern methods of using ice and rapid transport, that we are able to enjoy the benefits of fresh fish from the markets.

If possible, buy fresh foods each day. Supermarkets excel in offering very fresh vegetables, fruit, meat and fish. If you can grow some of your own, the benefits are enormous. "Organic" foods in shops although good , are often very highly priced. Also check the quality, they may sometimes be inferior to the "non-organic", if they have sat around on the shelves for days.

Cook at low temperatures.
If food is cooked, learn to enjoy it underdone rather than over-done. Steam food rather than boil in water. A steamer is a good investment. Boil the root vegetables that grow underground in the bottom of the steamer pan in the water, (keep for sauces) and steam the vegetables that grow above the ground in the top.

Cold pressed oils are best eaten raw or warm.
Frying temperatures change the structure of the oil molecules in such a way that they become more difficult to digest. If fat is kept and re-used, it can become rancid, burnt fat contains particles of carbon products. Both rancid and overheated fats are thought to be carcenogenic when consumed in quantity over long periods.

Cook dry, and add some melted butter or oil to it on your plate, which is much better for you when it has not been overheated.

We need oil in our diet for health. Use any of the cold pressed oils now freely available, use them cold where possible, or at the lowest cooking temperature possible. In some cases capsules containing evening primrose oil (which contains E.P.A.), may help relieve P.M.S symptoms, quite expensive but can be useful.

NUTRITIONAL SUPPLEMENTS

Do we really need nutritional supplements? Experts disagree as to whether one can actually get all the nutrients needed for health from the daily diet. In well trained expert hands, Applied Kinesiology* muscle testing is a reliable way to find out whether you need to take supplements to help strengthen your immune system, give you more energy, and keep you healthier. In nearly twenty years experience, almost everyone tested for nutrition seems to be deficient in some vitamins, or minerals, or both.

One thing is certain, extra nutrients are definitely needed when one has allowed one's immune system to become depleted, or when sickness or ill-health strikes. It is at these times, we really do need the additional support of specific supplements to supply the munitions for the fight back to health. If you have a problem with congestion, or a lump, then this is the time to take more care of yourself, and particularly in regard to your diet, so follow the suggestions on "foods best to avoid" on the previous pages.

Environmental pollution, and nutrient deficient foods are factors in uncontrolled oxidations. Oxidation produces free radicals which cause cell damage and faster aging. Our best protection is the anti-oxidant effect of vitamins A, C. and E., and the minerals, particularly Selenium. They all act together to prevent oxidation of each other. A protects C, C protects A, E, and B, and so on.

Vitamin A found in fish oils and yellow/green vegetables, is essential to the immune system and to protect the mucous membranes. You can also get Vitamin A and Vitamin E mixed with Selenium which is excellent. Too much A taken over a long period can become toxic, so follow expert advice. Beta-Carotene which the body uses to make Vitamin A, is even more safe as it is not toxic. A very large amount of Beta-Carotene may be taken for short periods when under stress or during illness. Most people are deficient of A in the winter, so make sure you are not.

For more information on Kinesiology, look in the index or write with S.A.E. to the publishers.

NUTRITIONAL SUPPLEMENTS

Vitamin B Complex is particularly needed in times of stress and nervous tension. If you drink alcohol a lot, or smoke, vitamin B is a must. The birth control pills tend to leach the body of Vitamin B6, so it is a good idea to take extra in tablet form.

Vitamin C is vital to health and our ability to fight infection. It is hard to get enough in our daily food. We need at least a gram a day to reinforce our immune system in these stressful times. The type of vitamin C tablets that contain bioflavonoids are best There is only about 25mg. in a large fresh orange, so we need to take more in tablet form. Also each cigarette smoked robs the body of up to 25mg. of vitamin C, so smokers would do well to take more than a gram a day as a rule, to replace what they lose.

Minerals are vital to overall health. Iron is for the blood. Choose a type that does not make you constipated. The "chelated" forms of minerals are usually absorbed better. Zinc for skin health, Chromium for blood sugar levels, and many others play a crucial role in our whole health picture. It certainly pays to take a good multi-mineral tablet daily. Dong Quai, an oriental herb, seems to help women who suffer from Pre-Menstrual Stress (P.M.S.), and the monthly "blues" very effectively. It may be a help to restore nutritional balance to the female reproductive system.

You will find that taking a course of vitamins regularly, with a break of a week every few weeks, then starting again, is a very wise measure for prevention. You will find you have less colds, catarrh and bouts of 'flu. You will fall prey to far fewer of those "bugs" that are always "going around".

Buying pots of supplements off the shelf is not necessarily the best way to tackle the problem, you may waste money. If you are unwell, or you feel you need the support of some additional nutrition, get the advice of a Kinesiologist, or another type of natural health care practitioner who has training in nutrition.

PREGNANCY & BREAST FEEDING

More babies are being born with defects, or develop problems at a very early age, than in previous decades. Why is this? How is it that so many babies, and very young children, now suffer from eczema, allergies, hives, and many other distressing complaints?

A child's health, and the strength of their immune system as it develops, is shaped by the start it gets from conception in its mother's womb. The mother's body is made of what she absorbs from what she eats, drinks and breathes.

Pregnant young women, and mothers with babes in arms can be observed smoking, and drinking alcohol in smoky pubs and restaurants. As they inhale the smoke, the tars and harmful chemicals are carried into the bloodstream, the same blood as is nourishing the growth of the unborn baby. It is the same with the alcohol. It is a potent poison in large enough quantities, and the tiny developing foetus is sensitive to all pollutants.

Many young women suffer from loosening teeth during their pregnancy because they do not get nearly enough calcium, magnesium and phosphorus in their daily diet, so as the baby grows, it robs the mother of her bone structure.

One way to increase calcium intake its to eat a plain natural yoghourt every day. Another way is to make bone stock from bones cooked for several hours with a little vinegar and a tin of tomatoes to provide the acid needed to help get the minerals in the bones into solution. This makes a wonderful stock as a base for home made soups, which are easy to make, and rich in the nutrients needed to make and maintain strong bones and teeth.

All the other dietary advice given previously is of much greater importance than ever when you are pregnant, or while you are breast feeding your young baby. Help yours to have the foods and strong immune system it needs to have healthy start in life.

PREGNANCY & BREAST FEEDING

An ideal time to make use of the preventive massage techniques is towards the end of pregnancy, and as the birth gets near. If you or your mate will gently massage your chest as illustrated, around the breasts, but never on the breast tissue itself, you may be able to keep your breasts quite clear, and feeling light. As your breasts become enlarged, they may feel heavy, or if they become congested and lumpy, you will find all of the breast decongestion techniques already explained of enormous value.

Wearing specially designed bras that give you the necessary support at this time is essential. Proper firm support will help you keep your figure by preventing undue stretching of the muscles and the skin of the upper chest. Once muscle tissue loses its original elasticity through constant stretch tension, it is virtually impossible to restore it to its original shape.

For some women, breast feeding their baby is a real delight, and for others a chore. In any event, breast feeding can be quite an uncomfortable procedure for the mother. It is at this time that it is most important to keep the skin of the breast supple and well nourished with oils. A Vitamin E oil capsule broken open, mixed and diluted with a vegetable oil, may help with cracked or sore nipples. This should be applied gently as soon as the feed is over, and especially after the last feed before you go to bed, to give the skin as much time as possible to restore itself.

Breasts can become congested during the months of feeding. Lumpiness and even mastitis can make the breasts extremely uncomfortable, and even painful. Nursing mothers who have used the "touch the breast and massage the outside of the leg" method, have been surprised at the degree of relief they have achieved. Even hard milky lumps can often be dispersed in a few minutes. One mother who uses these methods found that milk lumps may also disperse if you touch lightly the lumpy areas while the baby is actually feeding.

WHAT GOES IN - MUST COME OUT

Another insidious way our health and resistance can become eroded is by failing to eliminate the body's waste products. In this manual we are looking at everything which can in any way affect the health of breast tissues as part of the whole body vitality.

Constipation is a very widespread problem. Even among people who do not think they are constipated. It is true that people have different body rhythms, but most people would benefit from emptying their bowels more often. Not the most attractive topic in the world, but certainly one of the most important to health.

If we eat two or three meals each day, is it unreasonable to suppose that we ought to eliminate at least twice. If you support each end of a garden hose on a box and fill it up with water the water will stay in the pipe. But if you add a jug of water to one end, a jugful will come out of the other end. The water in the pipe moves along each time you add another jugful.

Although the analogy does not hold exactly true, it does give an idea. Each time we eat a substantial meal, all the contents of the intestines have to move along the digestive tract as soon as the stomach empties into the small intestine. Ideally one would have a bowel movement each time this happens, or shortly thereafter.

A large proportion of the population does not have a bowel movement every day, and this is still considered "normal" by many authorities since it is so widespread. Without being at all unduly concerned, it is good to work towards a daily movement.

A sluggish bowel allows detritus, and toxic materials to stick to the walls of the large intestine more or less permanently. The daily defecation comes from material that has passed through the middle of the clogged up" tube".

These toxic residues in your bowels can rob you of energy.

ARE BOWELS & BREASTS LINKED?

That sounds rather an amusing question, and yes, in a sense they are. Of course bowel health, or lack of it, affects the whole body, but since this book is about breast health, let us focus on that aspect.

There is a specific link between bowel congestion and breast congestion. The bowel is also referred to as the colon which has three main parts, ascending, transverse, and descending.The area of the side of the legs which is massaged while touching the breast, actually covers a series of reflex points which are directly related to the efficient function of the colon or Large Intestine.

The reflexes on the right leg are linked to the ascending portion of the colon and part of the transverse colon, and the strip massaged on the left leg is related to the other side of the transverse colon, and also to the descending colon.

Quite why there is such an apparently direct connection between the Large Intestine and the breast does not matter, the fact that it helps both during massage is the important point.

If you are an individual that does not have at least one bowel movement every day, then that is maybe something to look at very carefully. Give some time and attention to changing your habits. Your whole health picture can change if you keep your bowels moving in the best way for you. Many people do not have a daily habitual rhythm for going to the toilet.

Most find they can retrain themselves quite easily. It is best to go upon rising in the morning. Every single day when you wake up, make a hot drink, and go to the toilet. It helps to put your feet on a block to raise them a few inches off the floor. Sit for a while, and do not under any circumstance strain, just sit. If nothing happens, just keep doing this adult "potty training" until it does. It pays off handsomely in the long run.

THE VALUE OF BOWEL CLEANSING

Special herbs which gently clean out the bowels can enhance health greatly. Old faecal matter which adheres to the walls of the large bowel has a toxic effect on our whole system. It can be one reason why we never really feel fit as a fiddle. That draggy, listless, fed up feeling, can come from a clogged and dirty bowel.

Even if one goes to the toilet every day, virtually everyone has old material in the nooks and crannies of the intestine. If ignored this material can form diverticuli, or pockets of ancient stuff which stays there permanently unless it is encouraged to leave.

The large intestine contains pounds of friendly bacteria which help to process the contents of the bowel as it leaves the body. When there is a certain amount of old material present, it can upset the delicate acid/alkali, or pH balance of the large intestine.

If the bowel is allowed to become alkaline, unfriendly bacteria can multiply more easily and overtake the friendly population. This can give rise to an overgrowth of Candida Albicans and also provide a favourable environment for Thrush to develop. The Australian "Tea Tree Oil" can be very helpful for these conditions.

As long as this pH imbalance remains, Candida and Thrush are resistant to treatment and will return if the conditions in the bowel are not corrected. It is relatively easy to correct the situation with herbs. These do not cause one to become loose, but they do clean out the bowel very effectively, if taken continuously for several weeks initially, then from time to time for a week or so.

Bowel cleansing with gentle herbs can gradually dissolve away the sticky material which holds these deposits in place. Taking some specially formulated herbal combinations for a few weeks slowly but surely cleans the whole bowel up again. You may want to consult a natural health care practitioner, or buy yourself some herbs. They are formulated to be perfectly safe to take.

THE EMOTIONAL PART OF US
WHAT WE THINK, AFFECTS OUR HEALTH

There is a great deal of talk about breast cancer these days. And not without good reason. Women are urged to check their breasts regularly for lumps, or undue tenderness. This should be part of every woman's health care routine.

If a lump is detected, there is a natural reaction to be concerned, even alarmed. It is hoped that this manual will help dispel much of that fear, since almost all lumps, when detected early enough will respond to the practical self-help techniques described in the earlier pages.

The question remains, "Supposing the lumps do not go away using the massage techniques described?"

There is still no need for panic, or undue concern. The majority of cystic or fibrous lumps are usually benign growths, which are in no way life threatening. They can usually be dealt with in a very efficient way, and with very little disruption to the body.

But the fact remains, that some people get breast cancer. Again, the earlier any abnormalities are detected, the better chance there is of a complete cure. So it pays to be vigilant, and check yourself out regularly, but without a fearful concern.

In caring for our bodies, we can become overly concerned if we think that things are not as they should be. Fear and anxiety are very destructive emotions. Any condition of the human frame can be made much worse if fear is allowed to dominate one's mind. Especially is this so with any form of disease.

The "placebo effect" is the name given to the beneficial effect that our minds can have upon our bodies. If we think that something will do us good, it frequently does, even if the tablet or substance concerned has no known therapeutic effect whatsoever.

Experiments have been conducted with groups of people who had a given health problem. The groups studied were divided in two. One group was given the appropriate medication for the condition they were suffering from, and the other half was given a "placebo" which may have been sugar pills. Neither group had any idea what they were actually getting, but they all thought they were receiving the proper medicine.

In all these studies, a significant number of the people who took the sugar tablets showed improvements, and some recovered completely from their condition. Many such trials have been conducted, even with wounded men on the battlefield.

When the medics ran out of morphine, they injected distilled water into men who were badly wounded and told them that it was morphine, a very powerful pain-killer. Half the men so treated, said they got relief from the injections! Such is the power of the mind. Be positive about the health of your breasts!

If the placebo effect can help someone get better because of the power of the mind, then it is possible for the mind to have the opposite effect. Worrying about your breasts should be avoided.

"Psychosomatic" is a word which is frequently used, and it is also regretfully misused. It is frequently misused to convey the idea that the problem, whatever it is, is "all in the mind". Often when someone is told that their condition is "psychosomatic", it can seem to them to imply that they are imagining the condition.

This can and does cause great distress to some people, who know instinctively that something is really wrong. They may be worrying about it, perhaps even more than is necessary, but the fact remains that they know that something is wrong. To be told in effect that they are imagining it can be very hurtful, and even insulting.

The word *psychosomatic* comes from two ancient greek words, *psyche* meaning the mind, and *soma* meaning the body. It is a well known fact that years of excessive worrying can cause stomach or duodenal ulcers, that anger can aggravate high blood pressure. It is known that there is a direct correlation between destructive emotions and some particular diseases. In fact, every disease process has a mental/emotional component.

If you can have psychosomatic disease -
then you can have psychosomatic health!!

All good doctors know that just because a patient has had all the tests imaginable, and no recognisable condition or disease can be diagnosed with the information available. It does not mean there is no actual problem. Diagnosis is one of the most difficult areas of medicine. Many disease conditions develop very slowly in the body, and are virtually undetectable in the early stages.

The finest defence against disease is health itself. If we maintain a positive optimistic mental attitude, eat so we are well nourished, get adequate regular exercise, then health is the result. Health needs cultivating, it doesn't just happen. We need actively to cultivate a type of life-style that will produce health.

That does not mean that we have to become hypochondriacs, always worrying about our health and what can be wrong with us. Some people even study medical dictionaries and imagine they have every complaint in the book. Not a good idea! Nor do we need to spend our lives in health food shops and sports clubs in order to build up our health.

The secret is balance. Balance is needed in all things. Not too little food and not too much. Not too many indulgencies, and not too few either! A little of what you fancy really does you good! Not too much exercise, and not too little. A warm and happy disposition enables us to enjoy life more, makes us more loved and appreciated by those around us, and healthier too.

Lack Of Self Esteem spells *LOSE!*

Lack of self-esteem is undoubtedly the single biggest problem with human beings, men and women alike. Our self-image is a very fragile creature indeed. Don't be a loser!

When we are born, the birth trauma itself does nothing to boost our self-confidence. From a warm bath in a place with subdued light, we are thrust violently into a new environment of loud noises and bright lights, and sometimes a firm slap on the bottom! Most recover quickly from this ordeal as we bask in the adoration of mother, father, and relatives. Well fed, pampered, our every need attended to, we start to adjust to this new life.

Then we go to nursery, and the competition with others begins. The tears and frustrations of being put down starts. Then to school, with all its problems of trying to make the grade, getting on the wrong side of teachers, being at the bottom of the class.

It is not long before our parents start to criticise us, tell us we are wrong all the time, say we don't do this, and we don't do that, and why can't we be like that lovely little child next door!

We start to look at others, and see their shining strong points, and how much more clever they are than we are, and prettier, better dressed, nicer figure, higher grades, more boy friends, and we start to feel smaller and smaller. It is no small wonder that some social workers feel that by the time they leave school, most teenager's self-esteem is at a very low ebb indeed.

Each person is special and wonderfully unique. Comparing ourselves with others is unwise. We are ourselves, and nobody in the world can be that person as well as we can. Appreciate yourself. Be nice to yourself. Build your self-esteem by always concentrating on your good points and strengths. Read books on self-improvement, and be happy with being who you are.

ACCEPT YOURSELF
"JUST THE WAY YOU ARE"

Someone once said with tongue in cheek in a humourous vein: Women are never satisfied. They are too fat or too thin, their hair is too short or too long, too straight or too curly, their breasts are too big or too small, and their derrieres are too large or not at all! There appears to be some truth in this observation. It really is quite hard to find anyone, male or female who deep down really loves and appreciates themselves "just the way they are".

This does not mean we should be smug and self-satisfied either. Simply that as we grow, develop and mature on our journey through life, we do so in a spirit of self-acceptance rather than constant self-criticism.

Most of us spend far too much of our time talking very unkindly to ourselves: "I wish I hadn't done that." "What a fool I was to listen to him." "I'm so clumsy." "I'm so spotty, I look revolting."

We can change that. Listen to the way you talk to yourself, and ask yourself the question, "What would I feel if someone else spoke to me like that?" Would you not be upset, angry, ..more?

Start practicing loving and accepting yourself today for who and what you are. After all, in truth, you are all you've got! So your hair is straight, some girls with curly hair would give their eye teeth for theirs to be straight like yours!

In accepting and appreciating your body, (and *especially* your breasts) your personality, and your abilities for what they are at present, with a positive frame of mind, you can go to work on improving those things you would like to change. An exercise class, personal development group work, or perhaps evening classes to be more qualified. And meanwhile while you progress, love and appreciate yourself every day for who you are.

LOVE YOURSELF AND YOUR BODY

There is not enough love in the world. People talk about "love" a lot, but most do not seem to know the true meaning of the word. "Falling in love" is a mythical notion that defines a strong feeling. Nobody likes to "fall", it usually hurts. "Falling in lust" would be a more appropriate description in most cases.

True love is like a building. It has to be thought about, designed, and carefully constructed on sound foundations. What are the true foundations of love? The first one is respect. Love cannot even be present, or get started, unless there is proper respect. Self respect is the first requirement of self-love.

The second requirement in the building of love is acceptance. If we do not accept ourselves just as we are while we are in the process of growing, developing and maturing, we cannot truly love ourselves. It follows that we cannot show love to others either, if we do not accept them with all their faults and failings.

The third foundational footing for a beautiful love "building" is communication. How do most people you know communicate with themselves? Most are highly critical of themselves. "I'm such an idiot to do that". "I'm so clumsy." "I never get it right". Then this spills over into our relationships with others, and we find ourselves being highly critical of others. Saying harsh and wounding things to ourselves, or to others, tears down the "building" and undermines its structure.

People scorn at the saying "Every day, in every way, I am getting better and better at living my life" But what is wrong with taking a positive attitude towards our daily development? Or in rejoicing at the growth of others around us? You and your body are all you've got. Respect, accept, and communicate with yourself and your body every day, in a loving way. The more we grow and show real love to ourselves, the more we can give love to others.

DEALING WITH EMOTIONAL STRESS

We all have to contend in daily life with many circumstances and events which create negative feelings. Keeping calm and centred at times of emotional upsets is not easy. Everybody experiences emotional stress in life. It affects us all adversely at one time or another. Despite all our efforts to keep smiling, life's trials and tribulations sometimes get us down.

When knocked off our emotional equilibrium, everything seems more difficult to handle. Unpleasant jobs we would tackle easily, difficult people we can normally cope with, stressors we can usually handle all suddenly become impossible to contend with.

When the mounting stressors involve excess input, "too much to do" or "too many things at once", anyone can develop feelings of confusion and being "unable to cope". We can easily be overwhelmed by the sheer number of things we have to deal with. This state of overwhelm can be greatly relieved with the "Mental Stress Release" (M.S.R.) technique shown next.

Under excessive mental stress the blood supply to the brain can become reduced, and unbalanced between the front and back lobes. When increasing stress induces fear, the thinking part of the brain is "paralysed". When the body engages its automatic "fight/flight" mechanism, all the body's resources are directed into dealing with the crisis. Clear objective thinking tends to go out of the window until the crisis is dealt with. Regrettably our ability to reason and think can be clouded for long periods if we are in emotional turmoil, and the stresses are not resolved.

The simple, yet very powerful M.S.R. technique will help anyone face a problem no matter how serious. Most people can gain almost immediate relief from the anguish they may be suffering. Nothing could be simpler to do, for it is merely the extension of a natural gesture we have done all our lives.

COMMON REACTIONS TO STRESS

There is a common physical reaction to being emotionally distressed. People will often quickly put their hands to their foreheads automatically, when faced with a situation that is emotionally difficult for them to deal with. It is perhaps only a brief gesture, but as soon as the stress gets hard to handle, the hand goes to the brow.

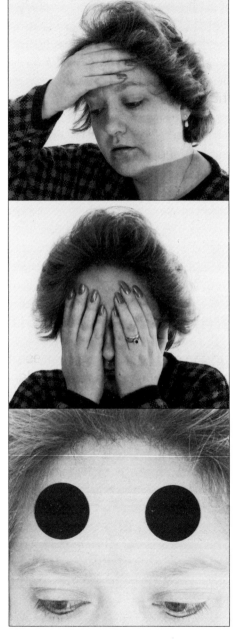

When people are very upset and feel tearful, they may often cover their faces with their palms. With both hands in this position, their fingertips may rest naturally on the two mounds on the forehead just above the iris of the eye. And without realising it, they are helping themselves to cope in a most remarkable way.

These two mounds on the forehead are called the 'frontal eminences'. The shape of the skull and the forehead varies from person to person, but everyone has these points. In some people they are very prominent, and in others with very flat foreheads, they may be quite difficult to see.

FIRST AID FOR MENTAL UPSETS

Although it may seem too good to be true, this gesture can be the key to relief from emotional distress. For instance, next time you have a shock or are upset, try this out. Place the fingertips of each hand in the position of this natural gesture. Use only enough pressure so that your fingers don't slip on the surface of the skin.

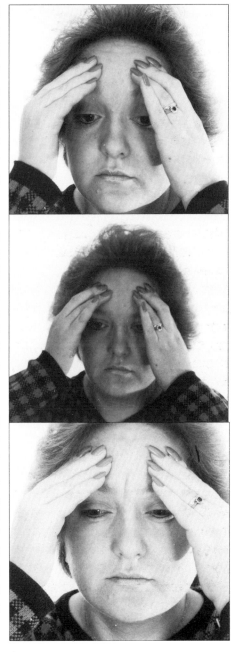

When this gentle contact has been made with the skin, if you maintain a very slight upward pressure towards the hairline, stretching the skin very slightly, just a millimetre or two, this is often even more effective. This stretch reflex appears to give some additional benefit.

Hold your fingertips steady in this position while you really concentrate hard on the very worst aspect of the problem. Within a short period of time, your feelings of distress will start to diminish. When held for periods of several minutes, this frequently enables even difficult problems to be faced much more easily and calmly than before it is done.

MENTAL STRESS RELEASE (M.S.R.)

The natural gesture people of touching the forehead is usually brief, only lasting a few seconds, and is ineffective. Our tendency when faced with life's unpleasant problems is to turn away from them, try to think of something else, or in some way to avoid the issue.

Using this technique while deliberately focussing on the problem is what seems to work best. The best results are obtained when the distressed individual maintains contact with the forehead for at least a minute or two. Sometimes up to ten or fifteen minutes contact are needed before relief will be obtained if the problem was of a serious or very traumatic nature.

Many individuals express surprise that their stress can be relieved so easily. A common response to this wonderful form of self-help is that often after only a minute or two, even the worst type of problems seemed to be of less stress or importance, or they say "it doesn't seem to matter so much" or "I just cannot seem to worry about it any more", or "it just drifted away".

On other occasions, individuals volunteer that a new possible solution had occurred to them which they had not thought of before. It really does help to get problems into perspective. It can be used for present stressors, or anxieties about future events or memories of past problems. Contacting these points appears to stimulate and balance the blood supply to the brain. A healthy blood supply is vital to clear thinking, free of emotional stress.

If you want to maintain contact with your own forehead, this will invariably have a beneficial effect. You can either use the fingertips of both hands, or cover the brow with the palm. However, it seems there is definitely an increased effectiveness when it is performed by another caring person. It is important for you, or for the person that you are helping, to concentrate on the core of the problem no matter how painful or upsetting this may be. So long as you keep your fingertips in place, the pain, distress and hurt will just seem to melt away in a matter of minutes. It is essential for the person to keep on focussing on the core of the problem, even if it tends to fade away, which it usually does. The wonderful bonus is that this effect is permanent.

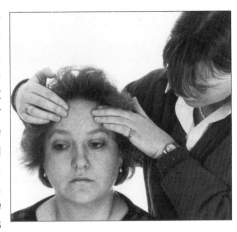

A further development of this way to Mental Stress Release can sometimes add even more potency to the effect. Place your left hand over your own forehead, or over the person's forehead, and with the right, cup the back of the skull. No pressure is required, merely a touch contact.

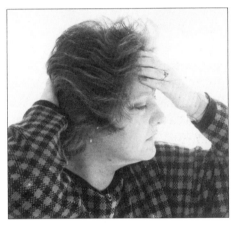

Alternatively, the thumb and fingertips of the left hand may be used as shown, with the right hand cupping the back of the head. This is often even more comforting than using fingers alone on the frontal eminences. Whatever it was upsetting to you or them will never again cause distress to

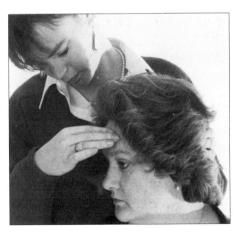

APPENDIX
WHAT IS APPLIED KINESIOLOGY?

What is Applied Kinesiology used for?
To help resolve the more than 80% of health problems that people suffer from that are not specific diseases; and for those who choose maintenance care, to enhance health and increase well-being.

Structurally: To alleviate back pain, aching shoulders, stiff necks, tennis and golfer's elbows, and virtually all structural problems.

Nutritionally: To discover causes for digestive problems and resolve them. It facilitates the treatment of allergies, and helps people to pinpoint their dietary imbalances and nutritional needs.

Emotionally: To give relief from mental stress, tension, anxieties, grief, fears, phobias and any form of emotional distress.

Energetically: In patients who are prone to chronic fatigue, post-viral syndrome, it is of great value in evaluating and correcting imbalances in the endocrine system. For those who are prone to fall prey to frequent infections, it enables assessment of the immune system of the body, and offers ways to strengthen it. Where disorders exist in the acupuncture meridians or other of the body's electrical systems, these can be addressed and balanced.

In short, the practice of Applied Kinesiology can help with all the health problems that plague such a high proportion of the population. In raising the standard of health and well-being, it ultimately reduces the cost of health care for the individual, and for the country collectively.

How is Applied Kinesiology used to obtain these results?
Muscles are gently tested to find where imbalances exist. The results are noted, and corrections are made in a priority order dictated by the person themselves in order to regain normal functions.

When the Kinesiologist locates and analyses the imbalances in the body, they are rebalanced with touch, massage and some nutritional support, which enhances the function of our internal natural healing processes. With regular balancing sessions involving muscle testing and some light massage on pressure points, adjustments to the dietary intake, and changes in lifestyle, Applied Kinesiologists find that most people enjoy a greater sense of health and well-being, and a reduction in the number of occasions when they feel unwell.

The development of Kinesiology into Applied Kinesiology

"Kinesiology" is the study of movement and muscle function. Orthodox physiotherapists many years ago devised a set of standard tests to check individual muscles and muscle groups to evaluate the extent to which their use was impaired after injury or strokes.

It is the practice of muscle testing, used by physical therapists to determine whether muscles were functioning correctly, the principles of which have been used for many years. The position for each of the muscle tests is shown in the standard textbooks on the subject. A highly respected text written was written by Kendal & Kendal.

Medical science has traditionally used muscle response testing for assessing certain bodily functions. When a light is shone into the eye, doctors observe the way the iris responds to the stimulus. In a knee jerk test, the leg is struck with a rubber hammer just below the knee to determine normal reflex action. These structural and neurological tests have provided the framework, and the basis for an entirely new method of testing, assessing, and correcting body functions.

Applied Kinesiology, (A.K.) was first discovered in 1964 by Dr. George Goodheart D.C., an eminent chiropractor in the United States of America.. It is an entirely new application of the principle of muscle testing. A.K. is a method of using the standard Kinesiological muscle tests, but applied to the evaluation of internal functions of the body. Applied Kinesiologists use the results to analyse how the person's body is working, and where functional problems exist.

Applied Kinesiology is an eclectic art developed over the last twenty-four years which embraces, utilises, and integrates the best ideas, therapies and techniques available from all branches of health care. It is a revolutionary new approach, which was much needed to cope with the ever increasing hazards of life on our polluted planet.

Dr. Goodheart's willingness to share his discoveries has led many vigorous and forward looking practitioners to investigate these new methods.   A.K. is now being researched, tested clinically, and new developments are being investigated by clinicians all over the world.

Applied Kinesiological muscle testing reveals systemic, structural and bio-chemical imbalances which can be rectified with many different techniques. Applied Kinesiology utilises technical information drawn from many different sources. This willingness to combine techniques from many disciplines has resulted in rapid growth and tremendous innovative progress.

Techniques, concepts and research from the world of Chiropractic has been blended with ancient oriental knowledge of acupuncture and the flow of energy in the body. Discoveries such as the reflexes of the famous osteopath Chapman, and the studies of the vascular system of the body made by the chiropractor Bennet have made vital contributions to the better understanding of physiology in action.

This new science provides a non-intrusive method of assessing the function of the various systems in the body. Using the muscle test response as a yardstick, the lymphatic system, the vascular system, the digestive system, among many others, can now be assessed using simple tests that are acceptable to the patient. These tests also reveal information about the intricacies of physiology previously unknown and unrecognised in the whole spectrum of health care.

Many patients have found relief using these methods. They have been thankful for the open mindedness which has led to these new discoveries. The new science of Applied Kinesiology is an effective tool which combines very well with every other form of health care.

What are the basic concepts behind Applied Kinesiology?
The most important basic concept is that the body has an innate knowledge of what is malfunctioning, and what may be done to correct it. Muscle testing can access some of this information, much of which the conscious mind is completely unaware of.

It is truly holistic, and the tests can reveal a picture of the many different types of imbalance that may be present in the individual. It can assess imbalances in all the aspects of an individual at the same time. The nutritional and structural realms, the mental stressors and energy pathways, that are each having their part in interfering with the bodies' ability to maintain overall health, are analysed together.

This "whole person" approach enables the Applied Kinesiologist to solve many obscure health problems that are caused as a result of an imbalance elsewhere. For instance, a structural problem with the atlas bone in the neck can be the cause of allergies. Allergies due to this cause will not be corrected by paying attention to the diet alone.

Another instance. An allergy to wheat could be causing someone to have panic attacks, which would not be solved by any amount of psychological help, until the chemical imbalance was addressed.

Who can it help, and what problems does it address?
The stresses and strains of life when excessive, cause some of the many systems of the body to go out of balance. If these minor imbalances are allowed to accumulate, eventually symptoms arise. Wisely used, Applied Kinesiology can pinpoint these imbalances and correct them, and in this way it is preventive. Almost all health problems are caused by compensations to physical, mental or dietary stresses. If minor imbalances are neglected over a long period, and allowed to accumulate, they lead to pain or feeling unwell, then later discomforting symptoms, and eventually disease can result.

Kinesiology offers ways to deal with all facets of any particular problem, and can offer help with a wide range of conditions. It can help those who have dietary problems, by testing for food sensitivities and allergies, vitamin and mineral deficiencies. Kinesiology has many ways to relieve or resolve mental distress, life-long phobias and fears, and even dyslexia can be helped.. Treatment is often successful in a matter of minutes, where conventional approaches may have taken months, and even then, only with limited success.

Conditions like lack of energy, frequent minor illnesses, and being generally run down is often due to internal stagnation of body fluids.

Kinesiology addresses this by balancing the lymphatic system which feeds and cleans the entire body where blood does not flow.

There are techniques to enhance blood flow with touch sensitive points located mostly on the scalp. Many people have chronic problems with digestion and elimination through the bowels. These may be normalised by the use of Applied Kinesiological techniques.

Muscular pain or tensions can cause postural distortion, leading to backache, neckache and other discomforts. These may be relieved using Kinesiological muscle balancing techniques which frequently reduce or avoid the need to move the bones in respect to each other with high velocity adjustments as practiced by some Osteopaths and Chiropractors.

Possibly most important of all, Kinesiology addresses many of the imbalances in the body's energy fields in a way which has never been possible before. All bodily movements are controlled by complex electrical circuits, much like computers. Applied Kinesiological muscle testing can reveal where these control 'computers' are out of tune, and correct them. In a very similar way to the motor car, if the electrical ignition system is out of tune, the mechanical parts of the car cannot run properly. It is the same with the human body.

So if the question is asked, "Who can it help?" the answer is "It can help everyone". Kinesiology not only provides a means whereby many distressing symptoms may be relieved and health restored, but by far and away its most awesome potential is in *prevention.*

Applied Kinesiology as a preventive tool.
You have already read in this manual how a simple Kinesiological technique can be used as a tool to help prevent congestion in the breasts from becoming worse, and maybe relieve it altogether. It is also a powerful tool to prevent a reoccurrence.

Applied Kinesiology in skilled hands can also help prevent the onset of ill health. When people are willing to undergo maintenance sessions, even when they appear to be perfectly well, minor imbalances can be discovered before they develop into something more serious.

By correcting these un-noticed minor imbalances, Kinesiology has tremendous potential in preventing the development of more serious health problems. It can harmonise and stimulate the natural innate healing power of the body. It helps people to become more health conscious, and take more responsibility for their own health.

It is often true that discomforting symptom patterns only emerge after many years of neglect or abuse. Preventive health care involving regular normalising of the musculo-skeletal frame, dispersing energy blockages and balancing the bio-computers, relieving mental tensions and emotional traumas as they occur, balancing the diet from week to week to avoid the onset of digestive problems or allergies, can only help to prevent disease, and enhance our enjoyment of life

Classes in Basic Aplied Kinesiology
Chiropractic assistants, Physiotherapist's staff, and others engaged in natural health care can learn basic Applied Kinesiology in a number of different ways. There are also special classes open to the general public who want to take more responsibility for their own health.

The author has written a basic textbook called **"Kinesiology and Balanced Health"** which is designed to give both the lay person and the professional helpers a sound understanding of the basics of Applied Kinesiology. The author was most cautious when compiling the book, to ensure that no technique offered to lay people could cause harm to anyone, even when performed ineptly by beginners.

It is a wonderful system of health care which has no side effects, but it is never suggested that Applied Kinesiology is all that is needed for total health care.

Basic classes for lay people teach wonderful things to help children learn and improve family health. Many hundreds of respected pro-fessionals, doctors, chiropractors, acupuncturists, dentists, osteo-paths, homeopaths, psychologists, etc., have attended weekend classes, become convinced of its value, and gone on to study it professionally. They find it can revolutionise the way they practise.

To find help from a practitioner, or for more information about Kinesiology and classes, write to the address at the back of this manual enclosing a large S.A.E.

IN CONCLUSION

Health problems are due more to life-style conditions than any one other factor. The argument whether environmental or factors of heridity are to blame for the human plight continues.

If we can kid ourselves that everything is down to heredity, and factors we are powerless to address, we have no hope but to submit to our fate, in which case any attempt to change the way we live is pointless.

An objective look at the world today must firmly place the blame for most of the world's health problems on the environmental issues. We certainly do inherit certain chracteristic weaknesses, and they cannot possibly account for the plethora of disastrous health conditions that extend worldwide. It is *how* we live.

This fact must be used to give us hope. For if we believe that the way we conduct ourselves from day to day does determine our future health, we will make the much needed changes.

This new science of "Applied Kinesiology", offers healing help never before available to aid the sick and deteriorating human state. The old proverb *"Prevention Is Better Than Cure"* has never been more true, and Applied Kinesiology offers a far greater potential for PREVENTION and more self-help health enhancement than any other system or health care modality on the face of the earth today.

The next decade will see the rapid growth of this "whole person approach" to health care. It will become a universal system. The idea that the local football team, or the Olympic team of the future will attempt to manage without an Applied Kinesiologist is nothing but laughable. You have seen a tiny window into the unimaginable wonders of A.K.. Find out more about it.
Tell your friends about this book, and let's help more people.

INDEX

INDEX

INDEX

INDEX